Compendium

The spiritual burning of incense
Basics, techniques, effects, and rituals

377 incenses for reference

Robert Mähr
Dr. Rodolfo Mähr

Imprint

1st edition 2018

English print edition, 2018

Verein Celecert, St. Gallen, Switzerland

Cover design: Moritz Mähr

Cover picture © Robert Mähr

© Celecert

ISBN: 978-3-9524898-3-3

www.celecert.org

Table of contents

Preface

How does one come up with the idea to publish yet another book about burning incense? Has not everything already been published multiple times? As it turned out during our research, there is one vast topic that has been neglected so far: the optimal burning temperature of the individual substances.

We came across this topic by accident. We had the idea to build a battery-powered "incense burning device" that would be fit to travel. When we defined the requirements, we encountered a simple question: how hot should this device be? As we could not find any reliable information in published textbooks or the internet, we had to deal with this problem ourselves.

During our first tests under laboratory conditions, with various temperatures and substances, it turned out that standardized procedures and substances are necessary in order to obtain comparable data. Whether one burns the fruits, the leaves, the roots or the resin is of importance. Besides, it makes a big difference whether one uses whole or pulverized plant pieces.

When we realized the complexity of the project, we started looking for possibilities to collect a maximum of relevant information with justifiable effort. We were aware that the results would never be complete – even if the title "Compendium" seems to imply a certain completeness.

The following circumstances make it difficult to classify collected data by order of to relevance:

- Empirical data, collected with analytical methods, only exists for some of the examined plant pieces.

- Traditional knowledge – so called "folk medicine" – is based upon principles that are hardly recognized today (e.g. the doctrine of signatures or humorism). Furthermore, the practices in folk medicine are often only comprehensible in the context of the respective culture.

- On the one hand, there is a lack of recognized and standardized analytical methods. On the other hand, the raw materials are not standardized in terms of content, origin or purity. A consistent naming of the individual raw materials would often already be helpful.

In this "compendium", we have combined all the information published in the referenced books with information from the internet and completed it with our own experiences and analyses. This approach is purely empirical and cannot claim to be complete. You, dear reader, are cordially invited to take part in the completion of this compendium. Maybe you can provide new insights or more detailed information which we will gladly incorporate into a new edition.

Finally, a word about our initial idea – the "incense burning device". Our research has shown that several of these devices are already available on the market and that they are continuously being developed and improved.

About the book

This book is the data basis for an app called Boswellia, which is being developed concurrently. Because Boswellia has been delayed due to technical reasons, we published the existing data electronically (Epub, Mobi) and in print (print on demand). This gives us the possibility to continuously be able to adjust the quality and quantity of our data with minimal effort.

About the authors

Robert Mähr graduated from the vocational school for rituals twelve years ago and has made a name for himself as ritual leader, master of ceremonies, and a celebrant since. Five years ago, he founded the Celert association with the aim of professionalizing ritual work and turning it into a recognized profession, comparable to the work of a pastor or an event manager. In addition, he works as an executive consultant, training manager, and project manager for companies and organizations.

Rodolfo Mähr has a PhD in cell biology. He has worked in both pharmaceutical as well as medicinal product research. He has also studied herbal medicine for over 30 years. He has collected or cultivated many of the plants in this book.

Introduction

Who was this book written for?

This compendium is directed both at beginners who want to learn the art of burning incense as well as experienced specialists who want to use this book for reference or to optimize the effect of certain substances and mixtures with regard to their temperature. A lot of previously published information has been collected and systematized. They are supplemented with our own practical experience, critically reviewed and, if necessary, adjusted or completed.

Definition

By "(incense) burning", we mean the controlled production of smoke by means of heating and/or burning one or several substances, hereafter called incenses. During ritual incense burnings, the emerging smoke is supposed to have a specific effect, such as cleansing people, objects, and places; strengthening mind and soul; improving general well-being; altering perception, increasing erotic desire; improving concentration or, simply, perfuming a room. Ritual incense burning is not a scientific discipline, even though it has been used for ritual purposes, and probably also as a form of therapy, since the beginning of humanity. It is a traditional practice that has spread and developed in all cultures worldwide. The therapeutic effect of certain incense essences is also acknowledged by orthodox medicine and is specifically used, for instance, in aromatherapy. The pharmaceutical, food, cosmetics, and advertising industries, and, of course, medicine have also taken advantage of the effects of the individual substances.

Where do the incense burning traditions come from?

This question cannot be answered definitively, as this tradition is known in virtually all cultures. It is assumed that people have been using incenses for ritual purposes since early history. It can further be assumed that humanity has a basic need to consciously use select essences for spiritual rituals, cleansing, and the healing of body and soul. People have certainly recognized the psychoactive effect of certain substances very early on and used them for "dream journeys" and spiritual cults. Since the beginning of controlled fire use, the cleansing of people, animals, and objects through incense has been verifiably practiced.

Areas of application

Unlike in Asian cultures, people in the Western world always burn incense to pursue a spiritual goal. This might have to do with the fact that the Catholic Church declared incense burning to be a spiritual or even sacred practice reserved for priests. In Hindu and Buddhist countries, incense burning is not only used for spiritual ceremonies, but also to disinfect rooms and objects and to drive out vermin. In the Western world, incense burning was used both for cleansing houses and yards as well as for healing therapies; and, as in Asia, it was central to daily life. To summarize, it can be said that there is actually no need for a specific reason to burn incense and that you can practice incense burning anytime and anyplace. However, it is important to keep in mind that certain incenses can cause unpleasant or allergic reactions (headaches, hay fever, rashes, etc.) in both humans and animals. Because of that, it is important to be considerate of one's environment when burning incense.

An important reason for the global spread of incense burning since primeval times is the fact that active substances are transmitted from the olfactory nerve (nervus olfactorius) to the brain within milliseconds. Thus, they have a direct and strong impact on the human and animal psyche. This factor was also used in primeval medicine, as there was no possibility to directly inject substances.

Incenses

Almost any substance can be used as an incense, but not all of them produce a pleasant and effective fragrance. The incenses referenced in this book are mostly used as medicinal herbs, generate recognizable and pleasant smoke and most of them can be found in retail. Hallucinogenic substances such as henbane, jimson weed, angel's trumpet, and others which cannot legally be sold in most countries are an exception.

When assessing the effect of individual incenses, it is important to consider that the quantity and ratios of the individual active substances may vary considerably according to the following criteria:

- Soil conditions

- Geographic location

- Genetic descent

- Microclimate

- Environmental conditions

- Extraction process

- Time of harvest

- Purity

Due to this diversity, it is understandable that a wide variety of products with equally varying qualities are sold on the market. Because this market does not have quality controls, there is, unfortunately, a lot of malpractice. Since antiquity, incenses have been mixed, adulterated, and falsely declared. Certain substances such as agarwood, frankincense, amber, and others have always been rare and thus very expensive, making malpractice very lucrative. Both for retail as well as for the layperson, such imitations are hard to recognize since our nose is often overwhelmed by these very complex aromas. Furthermore, they are natural products and can always display a degree of variability. Binding quality standards and appropriate controls would be helpful. Fortunately, a large number of retailers nowadays declare their incenses with Latin names, designation of origin and cultivation method, purity and potential effect.

Resins

Resin is an incense that is relatively unproblematic to handle because it usually dissolves into smoke over a wide temperature range. The hotter one burns the substance, the faster the resin dissolves and the more smoke it generates. If one burns resins on a portable hearth or a sieve, the resin, due to the low temperature, might liquefy before turning into smoke. Excessive heat can cause resins to burn, which is not desired and distorts the flavor and the effect.

Leaves

Leaves are usually burned as incenses in dried form. Portable hearths are very suitable for burning leaves because they do not get very hot and the danger of autoignition is smaller than if one burns them on coal. If leaves become too hot, they develop a burning smell very quickly.

Roots, wood, bark

The solid parts of a plant usually need a lot of energy to generate smoke in the first place. The temperature has to be raised very carefully so that the parts do not autoignite and a burnt smell will not overpower the desired aroma. When burning incenses on coal, it is essential to remove all burning residue from the coal.

Fruits and seeds

Many dried fruits can be burned without any problem and are part of the most important and prevalent incenses (e.g. tonka bean, fennel seeds, rose hips, juniper berries). In fruits with high sugar content (raisins, pineapple, currant, apple, and many more), the sugar caramelizes and produces an insulating layer, which prevents other substances from being released. Therefore, we have removed all of these substances from the following collection and advise you not to use them.

European incenses

Our native incenses have always been used as medicine, essences, and for cultic purposes. With the advent of synthetically produced medicine, the medical use of these incenses has largely been forgotten but is now gaining in popularity again. The tradition of burning incenses has, however, mostly survived in rural areas. Many plants that are used as incenses grow on our doorstep, which is why we rarely need "exotic" incenses. However, native plants often have to be collected and dried independently, as they are hard to find on the market.

Protected plants

In the past, some medical plants were collected extensively, and their habitat has been vastly reduced due to environmental influences. Hence, various plants had to be placed under conservational protection. As a rule, these plants may not be gathered nor unearthed in nature. More details can be found in national law and are based on the Berne convention (the agreement on the conservation of European wildlife in their natural habitats). Naturally, we commit to this protection and want to encourage our readers to do the same. To acquire these substances, we recommend purchasing cultivated plants or growing your own plants from seeds.

Non-European incenses

This term refers to all substances that are not native to and also have not been introduced to central Europe (neophytes). However, this does not mean that these plants do not grow in our region under special conditions (greenhouses, houseplants). Because these plants do not grow in the wild in Europe, they have to be imported. Some of them are sold under different or synonymous names. Unfortunately, import products often lack a certificate of origin or quality. Even though there is a clear declaration standard for the cosmetic and pharmaceutical industries, no such mandatory declaration standards exist for the incense market. However, some retailers declare their products voluntarily, and there is an increase of fair trade incenses on the market.

The following list uses, if possible, the Latin or the most commonly used name. Unfortunately, the sources are often ambiguous because many plants have been assigned collective terms or trade names in the literature. Upon closer inspection, "uniform" substances often turn out to be different plants. For example, at least three balsam tree substances are offered on the market under the name "copal".

Collection and preparation of incenses

When collecting incense plants, remember to adhere to moderation and not to gather protected plants. In many cases, you can buy seeds for these kinds of plants and grow them in your own garden or on your windowsill. We also advise laypeople to consult an illustrated plant handbook to avoid confusion (see bibliography). Collected plants should be dried carefully (avoiding direct sunlight, keeping them cool) and then be preserved as drily as possible. Storing them for longer periods of time is not advisable, as essential oils can diffuse even in airtight containers after a while, which changes their aroma. You can also create your own incenses, using coal and essential oils. Grind the coal with the help of a mortar until it turns into a fine powder. Put it into a sealable jar or cup and carefully drizzle the substance onto the coal. Approximately 50 drops are sufficient for a medium coal tablet. Close the lid and shake the container until the coal has absorbed the liquid evenly. The substance looks like a styrax but smells like the respective oil and can be burned very easily.

Different effects

We assessed the effectiveness of the individual incenses according to criteria from both science and folk medicine. Substances such as frankincense, hemp, or myrrh are not only important as spiritual incenses but are also used as therapeutics. In this context, it is also important to mention aroma therapy, which plays an increasingly important role in many areas of life. In malls, for example, scents are very consciously used to influence our purchasing behavior. Counter areas of banks are also perfumed with special scent mixtures in order to conjure up a specific image in the subconscious of its customers.

Medical effects

Over thousands of years, empirical and scientific research has recorded a large number of effects and side effects derived from the vast abundance of possible incenses and their active components. Oftentimes, the main active components were extracted from and developed out of natural mixtures. It has to be noted that with natural active components, just as with synthetic ones, every effect can be tied to secondary effects. The following list shows the most frequent and most researched effects of incenses on the human organism:

- allergy-stymying	- dehydrating
- anti-carcinogenic	- detoxifying
- anti-inflammatory	- digestive
- anti-pruritic	- disinfectant
- anti-rheumatic	- diuretic
- anti-thrombotic	- expectoran
- antiallergic	- germicidal
- antibacterial	- good for the skin
- antibiotic	- hair growth-stimulating
- anticoagulant	- hormonal
- antidepressant	- immuno-stimulatin

- antiepileptic
- antimicrobiologic
- antimycotic
- antioxidant
- antipyretic
- antiseptic
- antispasmodic
- antiviral
- aphrodisiac effect
- appetite-suppressing
- appetizing
- astringent
- bile producing
- blood cleansing
- blood pressure-reducing
- blood pressure-regulating
- calming
- carminative
- circulation-stimulating
- cleansing
- contracting
- cough suppressant
- decongestant

- improving the ability to concentrate
- intensifying
- invigorating
- labor-inducing
- laxative
- lowering blood sugar levels
- lymph-cleansing
- memory-strengthening
- mucolytic
- narcotic
- nervine
- pain-relieving
- paralyzing
- positively inotropic
- psychoactive
- relaxing
- soothing
- soporific
- stimulating
- stimulating metabolism
- virility-enhancing
- warming
- wound-healing

Effects in folk medicine

By this we mean the traditional effects which stem from observations of nature, self-experiments, and transcendental insights. Many incenses have also been used as "natural medicines" in the form of dietary supplements, poultices, infusions, or as ingredients in ointments in order to alleviate symptoms. Hildegard von Bingen described the inhalation of certain incenses to treat specific diseases almost 1,000 years ago. In folk medicine, incenses do not only have a direct effect on human beings but also on our environment, spaces, and objects. This view puts incenses into a larger spiritual context. As the literature describes very different and oftentimes contradictory effects, we limit ourselves to the following six main effects.

Protection

As incenses can have both positive as well as negative effects, it is possible to ward off unwanted effects of any kind with the help of the smoke. Insect protection illustrates this most obviously, as the burning of certain substances drives away unwanted animals. Figuratively, this also means that people can be protected from all "negative energies" with the help of incenses. For this purpose, incense is burned, for example, around ritual sites outdoors – a kind of symbolic fencing that protects a space from intruders. Indoors, incenses are mainly burned around doors and windows in order to ward off unwanted things.

Cleansing

Various incenses act as a disinfectant and often have an antibacterial effect. Furthermore, many types of incenses develop strong aromas that, through their perfuming effect, reinforce the subjective impression of cleanliness. We know this effect from the cosmetics industry and industrial cleaning supplies, which are often perfumed (lemon, lavender, cinnamon, etc.). This cleansing is not limited to objects and places but is also used on people that have been hurt emotionally or have been "contaminated" in a different way. As opposed to cleansing with water, cleansing with smoke often focuses on the psyche of the person concerned.

Strengthening

A big part of our mental and physical fitness can be traced back to our mental constitution, which, under certain circumstances, can be improved with the help of incenses. Selected substances broaden our horizon and strengthen us in our plans and intentions.

Eroticizing effect

Various incenses work as aphrodisiacs, which has been proven empirically and scientifically and has been known since the beginning of human history. The same substances are also used, among other purposes, in the perfume industry.

Feeling comfortable

Emotional balance gives people calmness and stability. The individual reaction to incenses and the entire environment plays an important role. Expressions such as "This feels good!" prove that a positive reaction is being triggered on an individual level.

Encounters

The encounter of people requires the inner willingness of both parties. This "inner opening" can be supported with the help of incenses, as there are often invisible but individually perceptible barriers between people (e.g. scents). Furthermore, scents can connect people through a shared history.

Concentration

Some substances directly affect our brain stem and improve our ability to concentrate and, by doing so, our mental performance.

Meditation

The burning of select incenses, such as nettles, elder, lavender, thuja, laurel, rose blossoms, or frankincense, supports meditation. Consciousness expands and for many people, it becomes easier to embrace a different state of mind.

Trance, dream, vision

A few incenses have a scientifically documented effect on the psyche and, because of that, their use is partly forbidden. These substances include, among others, hemp, datura, henbane, poppy, salvia, brugmansia or tobacco.

Transformation

In the Catholic and Orthodox Church, frankincense is an integral part of the liturgy and the church service and is used for various ritual acts (prayers, spiritual transformations, worship, blessing, and cleansing). These burnings of frankincense use, along with actual frankincense, mixtures of styrax, cinnamon, and rose for reasons of cost. In most religions, these incense burnings are used in spiritual rituals. For that purpose, copal, mugwort, salvia apiana, and agarwood are used along with frankincense.

Burning temperatures

The correct burning temperatures are, according to our experience, a central factor for optimal incense burning, as overly high temperatures can lead to unpleasant smells and can even be harmful to one's health. This effect is particularly evident especially when burning incenses on coal, as plant parts can turn dark brown and catch fire. In such cases, the temperature has to be lowered – for example by covering them with sand, cooling them down with water, or increasing the distance to the source of heat.

Finding the optimal burning temperature

The stated burning temperatures were determined with the help of empirical experiments using an electronically controlled, electric heating plate with a heating spectrum of 0° to 400°C (32° - 752°F). The temperatures in degrees Celsius are average values, which are useful for optimal smoke development. For reasons of simplification, only the temperature range of 180° to 250°C (356° - 482°F) was examined in 5°C (9°F) steps.

It can be assumed for all determined data that the different qualities of the samples (age of the plant, moisture content, size and location, time of picking, incense quantity) and the general conditions (outside temperature, humidity, air pressure) of the same substance can deviate significantly from the stated values.

Another reason for deviation is the different consistency of the individual incenses. Pulverized incenses generally require a lower burning temperature than bulkier plant parts; dried incenses generally require less energy than fresh plant parts.

It should also be remembered that when burned, many incenses undergo chemical changes. Oftentimes, an insulating layer of burned material (ash, cinder, etc.) forms on the side of the heat source, which has an insulating effect on the rest of the incense material.

The test arrangement was measured at 21°C (70°F). In practice, however, different outdoor temperatures, wind, or high humidity must be expected and can influence the result.

For many substances, higher temperatures (+ 20°C / + 36°F) only have marginal influence, as the substances do not change chemically but immediately go up in smoke.

Roots, leaves, bark, and wood often begin to smell unpleasant when temperatures get too high, which can transform the initially positive effect and sometimes even produce harmful substances. To prevent this, one should only combine substances that require a similar burning temperature in incense mixtures.

Measuring method

The pulverized or finely chopped incense samples or the resin of each individual substance were sprinkled or placed on the heating plate at 180°C (356°F). If there was no smoke, the temperature was raised by five degrees. This step was repeated until smoke was detected. The testers analyzed the smoke both optically as well as through their sense of scent. They also ensured that the incense did not smell burned or change its scent. Whenever this happened, the temperature was reduced by five degrees and the procedure was repeated with a new sample. In addition, they also paid attention to color changes (dark coloring) of the incense sample.

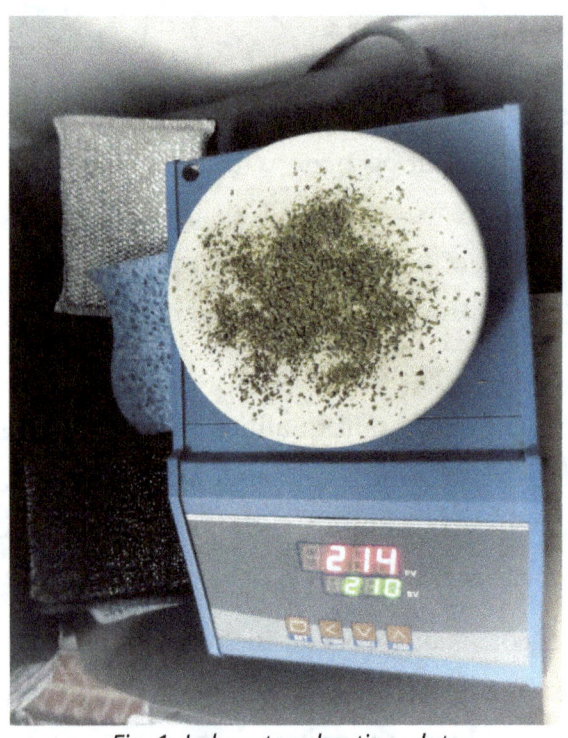
Fig. 1: Laboratory heating plate

This test procedure was carried out by the author for each substance and, afterwards, was repeated by a second independent tester with the same samples and under the same circumstances. In case of deviating results, both testers repeated the process until they reached a consensus.

For 20 randomly selected substances, control burnings with different plant parts (e.g. root and leaf) were conducted. No significant temperature differences were found. The collection of 377 incenses lists the optimal burning temperature for each substance.

Incense mixtures

Incense mixtures were probably already produced in prehistoric times; we know they have existed at least since antiquity. Mixtures from ancient Egypt (e.g. Kyphi), from Greece (e.g. zodiac sign mixtures), from the Arabic region (e.g. A Thousand and One Nights), from Israel (e.g. different frankincense mixtures) but also healing and protective mixtures from Celtic cultures (e.g. solstice) are well documented.

However, the interplay of the different ingredients with hundreds of active substances can trigger unwanted and sometimes uncontrolled reactions in our brain. Some incense mixtures contain substances with different burning temperatures. In order for the entire mixture to burn at the same time, substance which require low burning temperatures have to be burned at too high a temperature. In our view, this is not ideal because it can lead to toxic by-products.

Classic incense mixtures

Aegyptium

frankincense, acorus calamus, pistacia lentiscus, commiphora myrrha, commiphora, styrax officinalis, cinnamon

Afternoon of a faun

benzoin resin, cistus ladanifer, abelmoschus moschatus, geum urbanum, Indian sandalwood, styrax officinalis

Angel 1 (Berk)

angelica, frankincense, dammar gum, hierochloe odorata, Indian sandalwood

Angel 2 (Berk)

angelica, frankincense, eucalyptus globulus, cinnamomum camphora, mistletoe, citrus aurantium

Arabic incense mixture (Bakhoor or Bukhoor)

liquidambar styraciflua, frankincense, jasminum officinale, lavandula angustifolia, dog-rose, Indian sandalwood

Ariadne's herb meadow

dictamnus, cistus ladanifer, lavandula angustifolia, pistacia lentiscus, peppermint, sage

Aura protection cleaning (Berk)

amber, dracaena cinnabari, common fumitory, boswellia serrata, thyme, tulsi, common juniper, white sage

Avalon

frankincense, verbena officinalis, pistacia lentiscus, mistletoe, common juniper, silver fir

Ayla

Norway spruce, pistacia lentiscus, common juniper, silver fir

Blessing incense

commiphora myrrha, Indian sandalwood, styrax officinalis

Blue dragonfly on the lotus leaf (Summer Jap.)

commiphora myrrha, lavandula angustifolia, geum urbanum, Indian sandalwood, cinnamon

Breath of the Soul (Jap.)

benzoin resin, abelmoschus moschatus, Indian sandalwood, star anise, cinnamon

Busamé (The secret garden)

pistacia lentiscus, commiphora myrrha, nardostachys jatamansi, dog-rose, Indian sandalwood, cinnamon

Chill

eucalyptus globulus, sage, thyme

Chiron

iris x germanica, common myrtle, saffron crocus, sage, pistacia lentiscus

Cleaning (Be-Hozho-Na Ho Glachl)

hierochloe odorata, common juniper, white sage

Cleaning and clarification

frankincense, asafoetida, copal black, dracaena cinnabari, cinnamomum camphora, rosemary, sage, common juniper, Atlas cedar

Concentration

dammar gum, lemongras, verbena officinalis

Concentration (Berk)

alpinia galanga, cinnamomum camphora, pistacia lentiscus, geum urbanum, rosemary

Connection to primordial force 1 (Berk)

dammar gum, dracaena cinnabari, quercus robur, jasminum officinale, commiphora myrrha, common myrtle, vetiver

Connection to primordial force 2 (Berk)

frankincense, dammar gum, dog-rose, Indian sandalwood, styrax officinalis

Consecrated incense for the return of migratory birds

European larch, hierochloe odorata, blackthorn, common violet

Contact

frankincense, artemisia vulgaris, laurel, pistacia lentiscus

Contact with nature spirits 1 (Berk)

quercus robur, verbena officinalis, commiphora myrrha, common juniper, cinnamon

Contact with nature spirits 2 (Berk)

frankincense, artemisia vulgaris, alpinia galanga, common juniper

Don Juan (Kinkele)

cola acuminata, copal black, damiana, guaiacum officinale, acacia senegal , myristica fragrans, peppermint, balsam tolosanum, tonka beans

Dosha Dhoop (Kinkele)

benzoin resin, dammar gum, evernia prunastri, acacia senegal , acorus calamus, cardamon seed, geum urbanum, patchouli

Dream hummingbird

copal black, copal white, artemisia douglasiana

Druid

frankincense, fraxinus excelsior, pistacia lentiscus, geum urbanum, silver fir, cinnamon

Duir

elecampane, frankincense, artemisia vulgaris, commiphora myrrha, sage

Elemental beings

aspen, sage, marsh Labrador tea, common juniper, dog's mercury

Escape from ignorance (jap.)

agarwood, frankincense, geum urbanum, Indian sandalwood, cinnamon

Evening 1 (Berk)

frankincense, lavandula angustifolia, catunaregam spinosa, tetraclinis, Indian sandalwood, tonka beans

Evening 2 (Berk)

nardostachys jatamansi, commiphora myrrha, dog-rose, styrax officinalis, balsam tolosanum, tulsi

Fairy game

hierochloe odorata, elder, hop, pistacia lentiscus

First snowflakes in the pine grove (Winter Jap.)

agarwood, frankincense, cinnamomum camphora, commiphora myrrha, tetraclinis, cinnamon

Flight of the soul

frankincense, pistacia lentiscus, tetraclinis

Gilgamesh

acorus calamus, common myrtle, Atlas cedar

Gods' incense of the Mayas

courbaril, copal black, copal white, bursera graveolens

Golden jaguar (Mahucutah)

courbaril, bursera graveolens, sage

Good night

lavandula angustifolia, lemon balm, styrax officinalis

Greek temple incense

frankincense, amber, commiphora myrrha, Atlas cedar

Growing medium for phantoms

copal black, damiana, common fumitory, Norway spruce, ferula galbaniflua, guaiacum officinale, myristica fragrans, artemisia douglasiana, peganum harmala

Guardian angel

frankincense, dammar gum, pistacia lentiscus, tetraclinis

Guardian angel (for Simocho)

elecampane, dammar gum, fennel, Norway spruce, common myrtle, rosemary, tetraclinis, star anise, balsam tolosanum

Gullistan (The rose garden)

benzoin resin, abelmoschus moschatus, commiphora myrrha, geum urbanum, dog-rose, saffron crocus, Indian sandalwood, cinnamon

Harmonia

frankincense, coriander, pistacia lentiscus, commiphora myrrha

Harmony and creativity

frankincense, styrax benzoin, cinnamonkassie, lavandula angustifolia, commiphora, dog-rose, tonka beans, white sage, Atlas cedar

Healing (Na-Ho-Chldzl)

hierochloe odorata, white sage, yerba santa

Hopi

copal white, common juniper, white sage, sagebrush

House cleaning (Berk)

frankincense, asafoetida, copal black, cinnamomum camphora, hierochloe odorata, sage, common juniper

Indian cleaning

copal white, hierochloe odorata, white sage, Atlas cedar

Ischtar

benzoin resin, commiphora, Atlas cedar, cinnamon

Isis and Osiris

frankincense, commiphora myrrha,

Island of the blessed

coriander, cistus ladanifer, pistacia lentiscus, saffron crocus, star anise

Jaguar of the night (Caniztan)

courbaril, copal black, commiphora myrrha, balsam tolosanum, vanilla

Kailash (Tibetan)

alpinia galanga, commiphora wightii, cinnamomum camphora, Indian sandalwood, cinnamon

King David's seduction

agarwood, commiphora myrrha, Indian sandalwood, cinnamon

Kingdom of the angels

dammar gum, pistacia lentiscus, common myrtle, tetraclinis

Kyphi (Egyptian incense)

frankincense, benzoin resin, acorus calamus, cistus ladanifer, pistacia lentiscus, commiphora myrrha, common juniper, cinnamon, Mediterranean cypress

Lawudo (Tib.)

rhododendron anthopogon, common juniper,

Love

iris x germanica, dog-rose, Indian sandalwood, cinnamon

Love (Berk)

styrax benzoin, jasminum officinale, cistus ladanifer, patchouli, dog-rose, styrax officinalis, tonka beans

Lugal Banda

ferula galbaniflua, cistus ladanifer, pistacia lentiscus, commiphora myrrha, styrax officinalis

Lupuleda

frankincense, hop, scots pine, marsh Labrador tea, common juniper

Maneton

frankincense, alpinia galanga, acorus calamus, styrax officinalis

Meditation

frankincense, benzoin resin,

Meditation 1 (Berk)

commiphora wightii, Indian sandelwood,

Meditation 2 (Berk)

benzoin resin, bursera graveolens, styrax officinalis

Meditation and relaxation

angelica, frankincense, amber, copal black, verbena officinalis, eucalyptus globulus, laurel, Indian sandalwood, vetiver

Meditation in the evening

benzoin resin, commiphora wightii, Indian sandalwood

Meditation-smoking mixture

frankincense, boswellia frereana, commiphora wightii, lemongras

Mesopotamian mixture

benzoin resin, Indian sandelwood, styrax benzoin

Moments (Kinkele)

cinnamonkassie, ginger, cinnamomum camphora, abelmoschus moschatus, geum urbanum, frankincense, red sandalwood, star anise

Moon goddess

benzoin resin, boldo, courbaril, bursera graveolens

Morning of Bliss (Spring Jap.)

frankincense, cinnamomum camphora, geum urbanum, common juniper, silver fir

Movement and joy of life

frankincense, artemisia vulgaris, benzoin resin, tetraclinis, evernia prunastri, alpinia galanga, cardamon seed, red cedar, Atlas cedar

Nightlife (Autumn Jap.)

frankincense, cistus ladanifer, Indian sandalwood, styrax officinalis, cinnamon

Oraiba

boldo, common juniper, white sage, sagebrush

Phythia

dictamnus, cinnamomum camphora, cistus ladanifer, laurel, pistacia lentiscus, commiphora

Pink mystica

frankincense, cistus ladanifer, commiphora myrrha, dog-rose, tetraclinis, styrax officinalis

Plants of strength (Kinkele)

acorus calamus, stone pine, white sage, yerba santa, yerba santa, Atlas cedar

Pleasure of the heart

frankincense, benzoin resin, commiphora myrrha

Protective spirits

frankincense, scots pine, geum urbanum, common juniper

Raunacht (Rätsch)

amanita muscaria, cannabis, hyoscyamus niger, artemisia vulgaris, belladonna, Norway spruce, common juniper, silver fir, yew

Raunacht 1 (Berk)

asafoetida, artemisia vulgaris, common fumitory, Norway spruce, common juniper

Raunacht 2 (Berk)

angelica, amber, Norway spruce, hierochloe odorata

Rejection (Kinkele)

angelica, asafoetida, alpinia galanga, Japanese pepper, elder, ginger, liquorice, tilia, hyssop

Release 1 (Berk)

amber, common myrtle, commiphora, dog-rose, rosemary

Release 2 (Berk)

artemisia vulgaris, benzoin resin, dammar gum, alpinia galanga, balsam tolosanum

Sensuality and eroticism

benzoin resin, damiana, guaiacum officinale, commiphora wightii, ginger, coriander, abelmoschus moschatus, commiphora myrrha, cinnamon

Shakti

benzoin resin, commiphora wightii, coriander, saussurea costus, abelmoschus moschatus, geum urbanum, patchouli, Indian sandalwood

Shangri-La (tib.)

terminalia chebula, rhododendron anthopogon, common juniper

Shiva

dracaena cinnabari, commiphora wightii, saussurea costus, geum urbanum, Indian sandalwood

Sickness demon (Kinkele)

angelica, frankicense, alpinia galanga, lavandula angustifolia, commiphora myrrha, rosemary, thyme, common juniper, white willow

Soul

dog-rose, Indian sandelwood, balsam tolosanum, tonka beans

Steps of becoming

frankincense, dammar gum, juniperus macropoda, thuja occidentalis, abelmoschus moschatus, commiphora, rosemary, Indian sandalwood, star anise

Strength and clarity (Be-Ah-Dzill)

common juniper, lemongras, white sage, sagebrush

Temple incense

frankincense, ferula galbaniflua, commiphora myrrha, styrax officinalis

The blue bird

cinnamomum camphora, lavandula angustifolia, pistacia lentiscus, quince

Three royal incense

frankincense, benzoin resin, pistacia lentiscus, commiphora myrrha, cinnamon

Trust (Berk)

benzoin resin, jasminum officinale, citrus aurantium

Twelve holy nights

elecampane, frankincense, artemisia vulgaris, verbena officinalis, hypericum perforatum, chamomile, verbascum densiflorum, pistacia lentiscus, lemon balm, peppermint, sage, yarrow

Vision (Berk)

akashbeli, rhododendron anthopogon, mistletoe, shorea robusta

Wisdom and healing

commiphora wightii, juniperus macropoda, acorus calamus, scots pine, laurel, pistacia lentiscus, commiphora myrrha, patchouli, red sandalwood

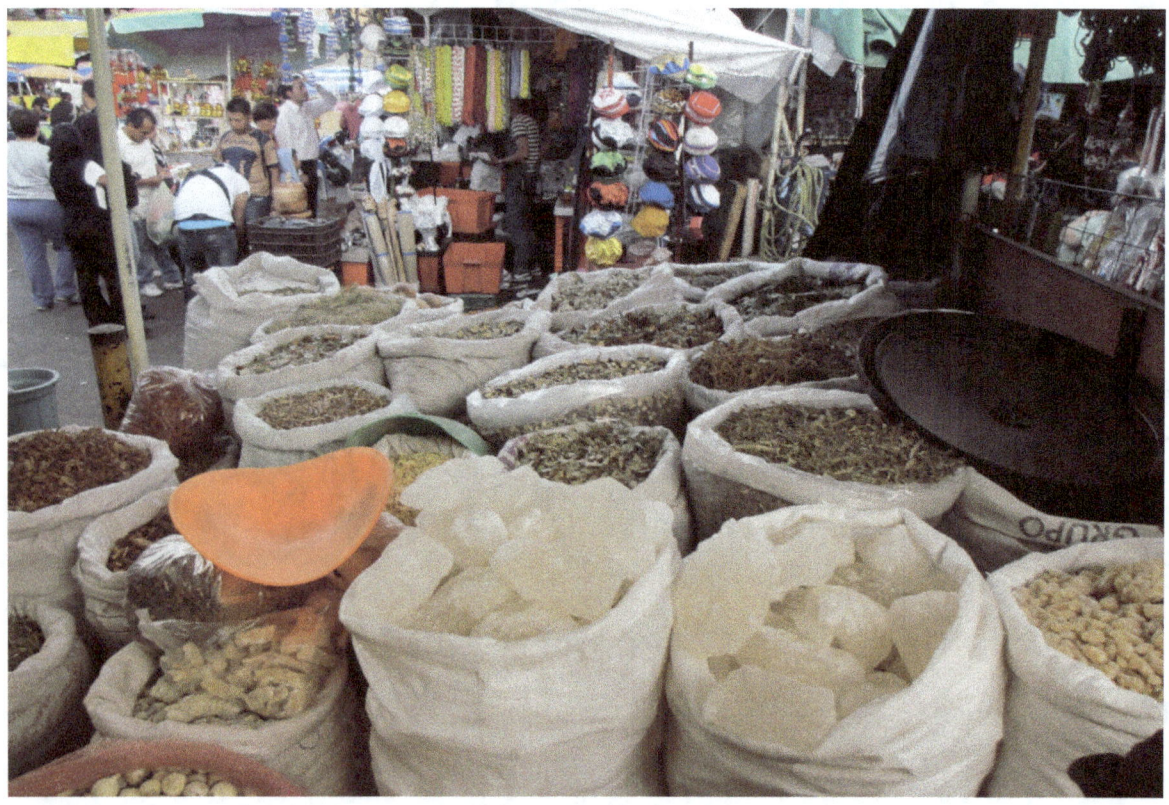

Fig. 2: Incenses Mexico City

Burning utensils

Incense sticks / cones / serpents / smudge bundles

A very simple and practical form of burning incense is the ignition of incense sticks and cones. Incense serpents, on the other hand, are not very common in Europe. They always contain the same ingredients that can, however, be used in different ways because of the different ways in which they were made.

Incense cones are lit at the top and then placed on a fireproof base. Depending on their size, they burn for between 5 – 30 minutes.

Incense sticks, often used in Buddhist and Hindu rituals, can be stuck into the earth, a container with sand, or into a special stand. They burn for approximately 5 – 15 minutes and are available in various qualities. Many incense sticks from India and China have a fine stem in the middle, which burns together with the incense and can distort the aroma. Japanese incense sticks and cones are different: they consist only of pure, pressed incense and do not contain any additives.

Incense serpents are mainly used in Asia to ward off insects, as they smoke very intensively and last for over an hour. They are either attached to special stands or placed on a fireproof base, such as a plate.

The disadvantages of these ready-made incense substances are the lack of aroma variety and the mostly non-transparent composition of their contents. For technical reasons, most incenses require additives (binders and adhesives) to be processed into incense cones, sticks, or serpents. Under certain circumstances, these additives can distort both their aroma as well as their effect.

Smudge bundles are a special and very old form of incense. Bound plants (e.g. mugwort, moxa, white sage etc.) are lit on one side and extinguished as soon as the bundle starts glowing. The smoke is then produced by swinging the bundle.

Incense vessels

The following list of incense vessels only shows some examples, as the individual articles only differ in appearance but not in the way they work.

Portable hearth

The most common portable hearths for burning incense are heated with the help of a candle, which guarantees a very stable temperature of 200° – 250° C and can be used for between two and four hours. These hearths are made from porcelain, stone, glass,

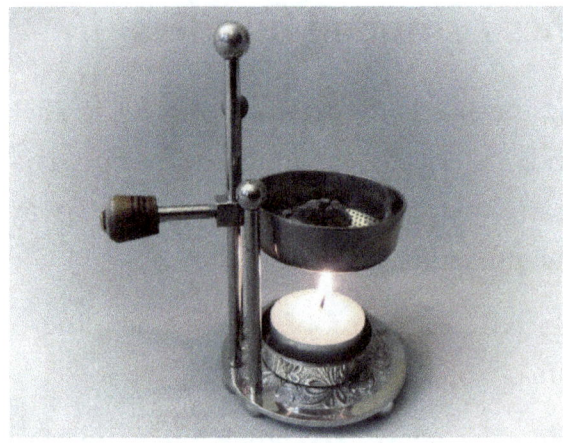

Fig. 3: Portable hearth

and metal and can be purchased inexpensively (from 20 CHF) on the market. Most models have a purposive distance between candle and sieve so that they can be used to burn incenses which require temperatures between 150° – 250° Celsius. Soft resins, such as dammar, copal blanco, larch, and finely ground incenses such as sandalwood, turmeric, or cinnamon, are problematic. When heated, the resins quickly turn liquid and drip into the candle wax, and the pulverized incenses can fall through the mesh of the sieve. In order to avoid this, aluminum foil or a thin sheet of glass can be placed on the sieve.

The market also offers portable incense hearths which offer an adjustable sieve or pan, which facilitates the regulation of temperature. With all portable incense hearths, it has to be taken into account that the candle, and thus the entire hearth, can reach a temperature of over 100° C. Caution must be taken when touching the hearth as well as choosing the base.

> Caution: fire hazard!

Open incense bowls

Fireproof vessels made from materials such as metal, stoneware, porcelain, wood or glass are suitable incense bowls. The bowl can be filled with sand or have suitable ventilation holes, so that the glowing coal does not directly touch its surface. This ensures that the coals' heat of approximately 300° is distributed more evenly

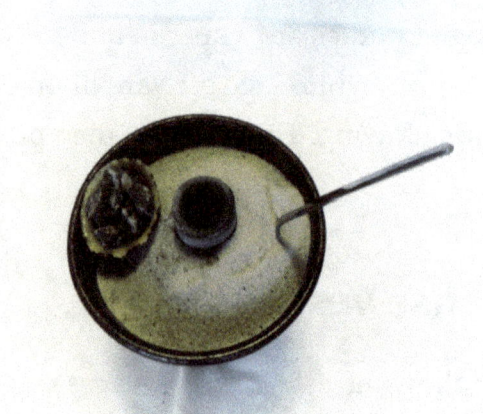

Fig. 4: Bowl, sand, coal, shell and spoon

and thus dissipates more quickly to the outside air, ensuring that the handles and base of the incense vessel do not heat up too much. Flat bowls are usually held in one's hand and thus must not become warmer than 40° C. To heat up the coal and to distribute the smoke, air is supplied by waving either a feather or a fan. Care has to be taken not to touch the glowing coal, so that it does not fall out of the vessel. Incense bowls are most suitable for burning incense outdoors but can also be used inside if handled carefully.

Caution: fire hazard!

Closed incense vessels

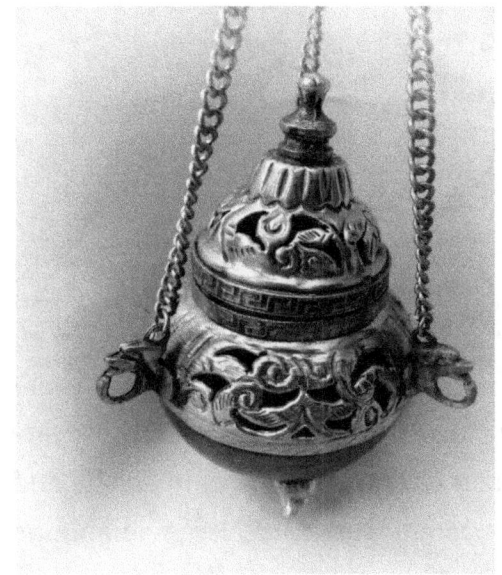

In both the Catholic as well as the Orthodox Church, thuribles are generally used. They are designed in such a way that the lid, after the glowing coal and the incense have been put into the vessel, is closed. Through swinging the vessel on its metal chains, a draft of air is created inside which generates more smoke.

In rural regions and all over Asia, incense pans are frequently used. Their handle is easy to hold and are used the same way as thuribles.

Fig. 5: incense vessel

Caution: When subsequently opening the lid, you can burn yourself on the hot metal parts!

Battery-powered incense burners

Since the introduction of e-cigarettes, battery-powered portable incense hearths can be found on market, which, in principle, combine all the advantages of the already existing incense burners. The temperature they produce is constant and can be regulated via a thermostat and they do not require an open flame, which reduces the risk of fire. Unfortunately, today's batteries do not provide enough energy to generate enough heat over a longer period of time. For certain resins these devices simply do not become hot enough. In addition, they are relatively pricey and can only burn small amounts of material.

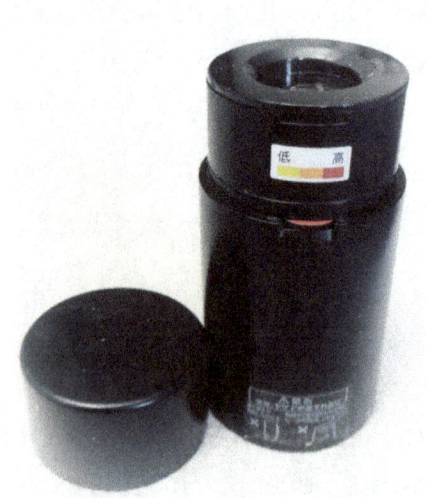

In Arab countries, people use electric portable hearths that can be plugged into power sockets in addition to traditional hearths. These devices are particularly suitable for continuous stationary use, such as the burning of incense in hotel lounges.

Fig. 6: Battery-powered incense burner

Coal

Incense burners require the same coal tablets as water pipes (shishas). These are manufactured artificially and offered in various sizes (25 mm – 40 mm) in shisha and tobacco shops. Natural coal and cubes of pressed camel dung are also available on the market. The rule that all coal must be burned until it no longer gives off its own taste applies to all products. Regular coal tablets are ready for use in just a few minutes. Natural coal takes a bit longer until it is truly hot. Coal products that have been exposed to air for a longer period of time might absorb moisture and become less flammable. That is why coal tablets should always be wrapped in aluminum foil or plastic bags. For incenses that require low burning temperatures (180°- 220°), one can pour some sand onto the glowing coal with the help of a spoon to reduce the temperature.

> Caution: As the coal heats up to over 200°C (392°F), it must not under any circumstances come into contact with skin or flammable materials. Special pliers, tweezers, and spoons should be used to move glowing coal!

Helpful little appliances

Flare matches are particularly suitable for lighting coal, as they produce an intense and extremely hot flame. Even in cold and strong winds, these lighters work perfect-

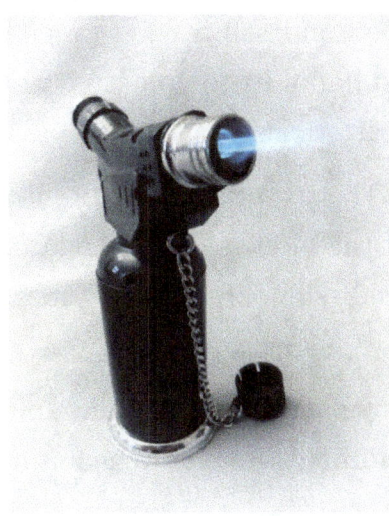

ly. Large bird feathers and fans lend themselves to making the coal glow even more and to distributing the smoke more evenly. If one wants to move around the room with the incense burner, the question of where to put the additional incense material arises. Shells, which are placed at the edge of the burning vessel, lend themselves to this purpose. One can remove the smoke residue from the coal and add new incense material with the help of a small spoon. Special metal tongs are required to handle glowing coal.

Fig. 7: Flare match

For safety reasons, only fireproof objects may be used.

Starter set

Specialized stores offer complete incense-burning sets. These consist of:

Set A: a portable hearth with a candle and an assortment of incenses.

Set B: an incense bowl, coal, sand, and an assortment of incenses.

The question is: which set is more suitable for beginners? In order to answer this question, you first have to know where and for what purpose you want to burn incense. For burning incense indoors, we recommend set A, even though it is also possible to use set B in indoor spaces. We recommend set B for outdoor use, because the candle of the portable hearth is sensitive to draughts and will not produce a lot of smoke.

Sources of supply

You can gather incense materials in nature and thus produce them yourself. Howe-ver, this only works for native incense substances and is mainly possible in spring and summer. Thus, one is often dependent on retailers. Apart from official and certified retailers such as pharmacies and drugstores, there are a large number of suppliers with partly questionable products of unclear origin and without a quality certificate. Impure and imitated materials often cannot be recognized by laypeople.

Specialized esoteric shops are usually very well assorted and sell a wide range of incenses and accessories. They also offer competent consultations and you can try out special substances in the store, which justifies their steeper pricing.

Many bookstores have an "esoteric corner" nowadays. Their supply is usually very limited and they do not provide customer consultation. The incense utensils on offer are often unusable and can only be used for decoration at best, not for burning incense.

You can find anything on the internet, including, of course, any kind of incense burning utensils. Here it is important once again to find a legitimate retailer, which is not easy due to the lack of quality certificates (see appendix).

When purchasing incenses online, you have to ensure that the substances on offer can be imported legally. Abroad, you can buy incenses on large, specialized markets (e.g. bazaars, souks, etc.). Here it is also important to be skeptical and to negotiate the price, as vendors often sell overpriced products of poor quality to tourists. To make sure that you are buying the right product, you should test it before you buy it; usually you can rely on your nose.

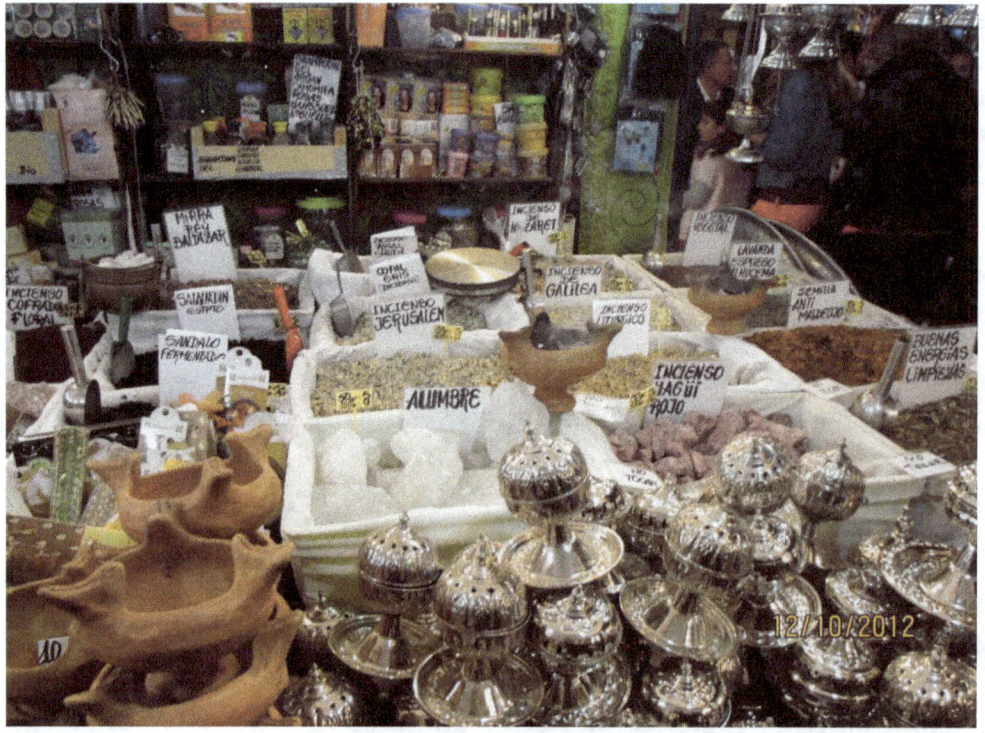

Fig. 8: Market in Granada (Spain)

Practical tips for incense burning

There is no correct or wrong way of burning incense, as every person has to burn incense in a way that is right for them. This means that there are situations in which you can or have to improvise with the supplies available and within the given framework. The following descriptions provide insight into commonly used tools and methods as well as advice and instructions that have proven themselves handy in practice.

Burning incense indoors

For burning incense indoors, closed and electric incense bowls and portable hearths are most suitable because they are safe and easy to use. Since they do not provide enough heat for certain substances, cannot be swung around, and oftentimes do not emit enough smoke, open incense bowls are also a possibility if handled carefully.

Both modern rooms as well as many old buildings are now equipped with smoke alarms that even react to the faintest bit of smoke.

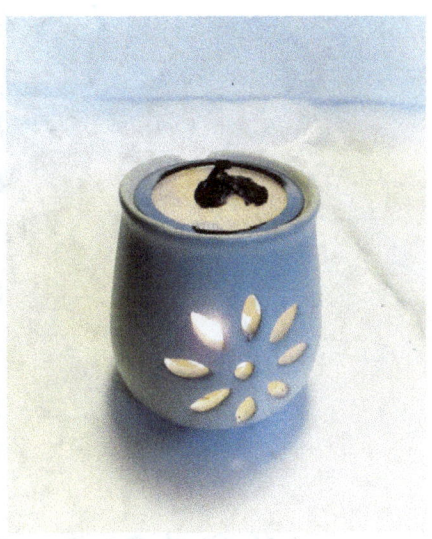

Fig. 9: Stone incense burner

The fire protection systems have to be deactivated and reactivated afterwards.

Burning incense outdoors

Outdoors, the wind and the weather always have to be taken into account, which is why incense bundles or coal are most often used. They are used in both closed as well as open incense burners. The shape and type of the incense burner is usually determined by tradition. Native American and shamanic incense rituals use stone and pottery bowls, shells, chalices or wooden vessels. The church, on the other hand, prefers closed thuribles. Farmers mostly used old pans to burn incense in their yards and stables. Even though there are no almost limits to the variety of incense burners, you should test their usefulness beforehand. The following points have to be taken into account:

> Touching the vessel might cause burns.
> The heat source (coal, candle) must not fall out when swinging.
> The embers need oxygen to keep them from going out.

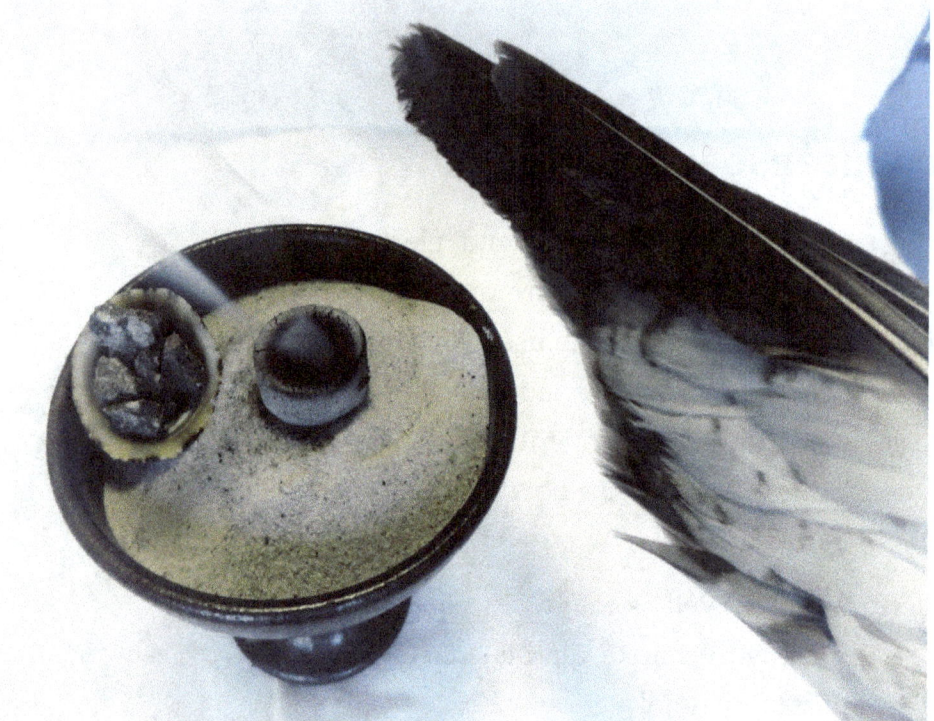

Fig. 10: Smoking with bussard feather

Incense burning techniques in other cultures

Due to differing climate conditions and the varying materials available, different cultures developed different burning techniques. The worldwide spread of Catholicism has led to the replacement of traditional burning techniques by ecclesiastical incense burning in many countries.

Native American and shamanic techniques

The most well-known Native American incense-burning technique is the burning of smudge bundles of white sage or prairie mugwort. It can be assumed that this type of incense-burning stems from prehistoric times, as it requires hardly any resources other than fire. All it takes is a bundle of the incense plant and a fire to light it. A shared fire was of central importance in these cultures, which is why they must have burned incenses on open fires. Burning incense on glowing rocks, as it is practiced, for example, in sweat lodges, is also widespread. The indigenous peoples of North, Central, and South America also burn incense in open incense bowls made from stone, shells, or wood. To spread the smoke, they usually use rare bird feathers, fans made from feathers or bark, and tufts of plants.

Oriental incense burning

The Orient generally uses resin (e.g. frankincense, myrrh, hashish) and traditional incense mixtures. The choice of incense mainly has to do with the preservability of these substances. The climate-induced heat does not affect the resins, even if they are stored for a long time. On the contrary: these substances become even more long-lasting and sometimes refined in their aroma. Portable hearths, special lamps and pans are used for burning incense. People in the Orient also use coal or dried manure in open vessels.

Incense burning techniques in Asia

Throughout Asia, people burn a large amount of incense, and in some countries it is even part of their everyday lives. For that purpose, people mainly use incense serpents and cones as well as incense snails. The advantage of this technique is that it is uncomplicated and inexpensive. Incense sticks are used in both Hindu as well as Buddhist praying rituals, which means that they are omnipresent. In Buddhist temples, incense sticks are even burned in bundles together with their packaging in special "ovens". It goes without saying that the quality of the aroma only plays a minor role. The Japanese have developed high-quality incense sticks which contain hardly any additives. They are mainly used for Buddhist rituals.

Modern incense burning techniques

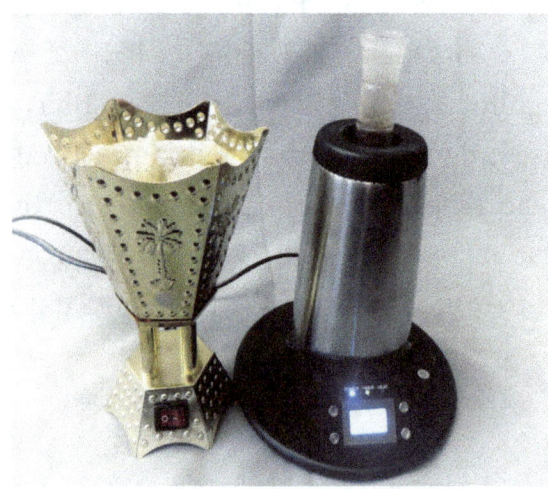

Fig. 11: Modern incense burners

In addition to the traditional incense burning techniques mentioned above, electric devices and evaporators are also used today. People also use electric coal which was developed for heating water pipes and can be connected to a socket. When used to burn incense, however, electric coal has various disadvantages: due to its connection to the socket, it can only be used stationaryily, and it cannot precisely regulate temperatures. To overcome these disadvantages, battery-powered portable hearths are also used. However, the devices we tested did not stand up to comparison with height-adjustable portable hearths that include a candle. Although they do allow for temperature regulation, their heating capacity is unfortunately too low to burn larger quantities of incenses.

Incense burning rituals

The following collection of common incense-burning rituals is not exhaustive. The descriptions should also not be understood as rigid procedures. They are suggestions on how to use incense in practice. Readers should be inspired to develop and try out their own forms and variations in order to adapt these rituals to their own contexts. Participants, place, time, and aim play an important role. These adaptations allow for new forms and variations of traditional rituals. Rituals must be transparent and voluntary, and this general rule also applies to the rituals listed below. Likewise, the appropriate safety measures must be taken into account.

Cleansing people

Many people feel uncomfortable "in their skin" after certain situations, encounters, and visits to contaminated places. This feeling is even stronger if people are touched or harmed. Through the burning of incense, the affected people can overcome this threatening or painful feeling – or its impact can at least be reduced. Figuratively, the soul is cleansed.

First of all, the affected person selects the appropriate incense and the right place. Then the person for whom the incense is burned stands with their legs slightly apart so that the person who burns the incense has enough room to move around them. When the incense is burned, it makes sense for the affected person to close their eyes in order to avoid any distractions. Cleansing usually starts at the head and moves towards the ground. There are no limits to your imagination – as long as the other person feels at ease.

This ritual takes about 5 – 15 minutes.

Burning incense in houses

Burning incense in new and/or renovated buildings is an ancient tradition. In practice, this tradition neutralizes the smells of building materials and the people who have worked in these rooms. It is a classic cleansing ritual. On the other hand, this ritual also constitutes a marking of the new inhabitants and the occupation of this «new» place.

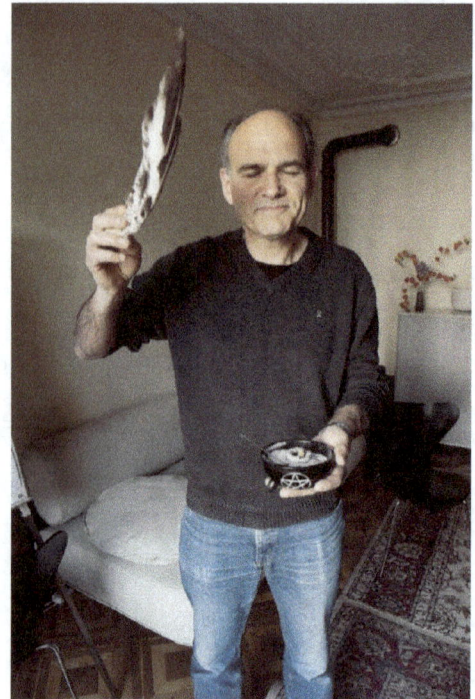

Fig. 12: Traditional "Hausräuke"

The burning of incense in houses is usually carried out by the residents themselves. Everyone individually selects a suitable substance or mixture and burns it according to their preference within their rooms. Shared rooms are usually cleansed together.

If guests are present, they should withdraw from the rooms when the incense is burned so as not to disturb the intimacy. If needed, they can be encouraged to support the new residents in their plans by focusing their energy through music, singing, or concentration. This ritual usually takes about 10 – 30 minutes. It should under no circumstances take too long, so that the thoughts of the guests do not stray. For those guests who do not wish to participate, an alternative program should be offered. After this contemplative act, the usual festivities (breaking bread, delivering blessings, building rituals, etc.) can be held.

Cleansing rooms and places

Certain places can be contaminated, either by odors or by other disturbing energies that sensitive people can perceive negatively. The use of cleansing incenses can create a positive, or at least a neutral atmosphere. This type of incense-burning is often used in preparation of events. Care must therefore be taken to ensure that the incense does not cause unwanted feelings in the participants. In this context, for example, frankincense and white sage must be handled with caution, because frankincense reminds Catholics and ex-Catholics of the church, and white

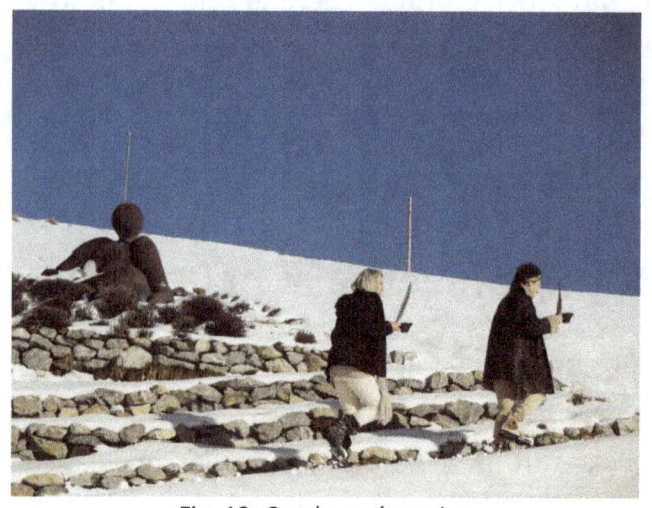

Fig. 13: Outdoor cleansing

sage is often associated with Native American rituals. After incense burnings, rooms may have to be ventilated to neutralize the smell.

Inaugural incense-burning

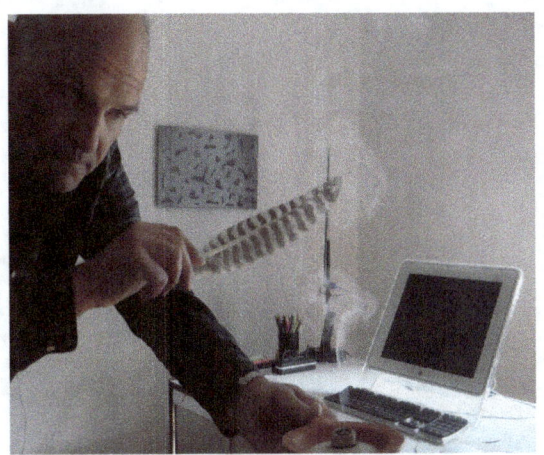
Fig. 14: Office cleansing

Incense-burning can be used to inaugurate projects, events or other works. It does not matter whether the incense is burned in the presence of the work itself or just a symbolic representation of the work. This ritual is also about cleansing as well as the appreciation and spreading of positive energy that is passed on through the inauguration ritual. A similar ritual is practiced by the Catholic Church under the name of 'blessing'.

Burning incense as a farewell ritual

With the burning of select substances, memories can be retrieved and linked to special moments. These two effects are used in farewell rituals. Smoke, as a transient state of matter, is a fitting symbol for the end, for letting go and saying farewell. The right incense or mixture can enable a connection with the things to come and a reconciliation with problems of the past. Farewells and letting go are always the beginning of something new. Burning incense is often part of farewell rituals in which, for example, objects are burned, buried, or given to the water.

Ritual preparation

Incense rituals must be well prepared. Supplies have to be ready at the right time and in the right place. The assistance of other people is often helpful, so that the ritual does not take up too much time. Rituals that are too long can be strenuous for the participants, which can negatively influence their concentration and the overall effect. Rituals, minus framework program, should take between 10 and a maximum of 40 minutes. Again, the simple rule is that every ritual has to be transparent and voluntary.

Incense from A to Z

abata cola

LATIN	Cola acuminata (Schott & Endl.)
SYNONYMS	cola nut
SPREAD	Africa, South America
PLANT PARTS	fruits, nuts
TEMPERATURE	240°C / 464°F
SUBSTANCES	alkaloids, tanning agent, minerals
MEDICAL EFFECTS	stimulating
FOLK MEDICINE	eroticizing effect, encounters

absinthe

LATIN	Artemisia absinthium (L.)
SYNONYMS	absinth wormwood, absinthium
SPREAD	Africa, Asia, Europe, North America
PLANT PARTS	herb
TEMPERATURE	220°C / 428°F
SUBSTANCES	essential oils, flavonoids
MEDICAL EFFECTS	appetitstimulating, antispasmodic, digestive
FOLK MEDICINE	protection, eroticizing effect, meditation, transformation

African rue

LATIN	Peganum harmala (L.)
SYNONYMS	wild rue, Syrian rue, aspand, harmal
SPREAD	Africa, Asia, Europe, North America
PLANT PARTS	fruits, seeds
TEMPERATURE	205°C / 401°F
SUBSTANCES	alkaloids, essential oils
MEDICAL EFFECTS	psychoactive
FOLK MEDICINE	protection, trance, dream, vision , meditation, encounters

agar wood

LATIN	Aquilaria malaccensis (Lam.)
SYNONYMS	oud,oodh, agar, aloeswood, lign-aloes, gharuwood
SPREAD	Asia, Europe
PLANT PARTS	leaves, grains, root
TEMPERATURE	250°C / 482°F
SUBSTANCES	essential oils, flavonoids
MEDICAL EFFECTS	calming, mucolytic
FOLK MEDICINE	concentration, meditation, eroticizing effect, feeling comfortable
NOTES	There are different qualities (A-D), all in the upper price range. Since agarwood is extremely expensive, fakes are often sold.

agrimony

LATIN	Agrimonia eupatoria (L.)
SYNONYMS	common agrimony, church steeples, sticklewort
SPREAD	Asia, Europe
PLANT PARTS	herb
TEMPERATURE	225°C / 437°F
SUBSTANCES	essential oils, flavonoids, tanning agent, silica
MEDICAL EFFECTS	antiviral, anti-inflammatory
FOLK MEDICINE	meditation, transformation

akashbeli

LATIN	according to Dr. Chr. Rätsch not clearly assigned
SYNONYMS	
SPREAD	Asia
PLANT PARTS	wood
TEMPERATURE	220°C / 428°F
SUBSTANCES	essential oils
MEDICAL EFFECTS	calming
FOLK MEDICINE	meditation
NOTES	ref. Dr. Christian Rätsch, Germany

alfalfa

LATIN	Medicago sativa (L.)
SYNONYMS	sickle alfalfa, sickle medick, yellow lucerne, yellow alfalfa
SPREAD	Africa, Asia, Europe, North America, Oceania, South America
PLANT PARTS	herb
TEMPERATURE	225°C / 437°F
SUBSTANCES	coumarins, saponins, acids
MEDICAL EFFECTS	diuretic
FOLK MEDICINE	encounters, concentration, transformation

allspice

LATIN	Pimenta dioica (Merr.)
SYNONYMS	Jamaica pepper, pepper, myrtle pepper, pimenta, Turkish yenibahar, newspice
SPREAD	Africa, Asia, Oceania, South America
PLANT PARTS	leaves, grains, seeds
TEMPERATURE	230°C / 446°F
SUBSTANCES	essential oils
MEDICAL EFFECTS	antimicrobiologic
FOLK MEDICINE	protection, concentration, feeling comfortable
NOTES	toxic

aloe vera

LATIN	Aloe barbadensis (Mill.)
SYNONYMS	
SPREAD	Africa, Asia, Europe, North America, Oceania, South America
PLANT PARTS	resin
TEMPERATURE	230°C / 446°F (max. 250°C / 482°F)
SUBSTANCES	anthranoids, acids
MEDICAL EFFECTS	laxative, anti-inflammatory, immuno-stimulating, wound-healing
FOLK MEDICINE	concentration, feeling comfortable

alpine-rose

LATIN	Rhododendron ferrugineum (L.)
SYNONYMS	snow-rose, rusty-leaved alpenrose
SPREAD	Europe
PLANT PARTS	leaves
TEMPERATURE	215°C / 419°F
SUBSTANCES	essential oils, glycosides
MEDICAL EFFECTS	diuretic
FOLK MEDICINE	concentration
NOTES	protected plant

amber

LATIN	Coniferopsida
SYNONYMS	resinite
SPREAD	Africa, Asia, Europe, North America, Oceania, South America
PLANT PARTS	resin
TEMPERATURE	300°C / 572°F (and more)
SUBSTANCES	essential oils
MEDICAL EFFECTS	immuno-stimulating
FOLK MEDICINE	strengthening, meditation

American juniper

LATIN	Juniperus virginiana (L.)
SYNONYMS	eastern redcedar, Virginian juniper, red juniper, pencil cedar, aromatic cedar
SPREAD	North America
PLANT PARTS	leaves, fruits
TEMPERATURE	215°C / 419°F
SUBSTANCES	essential oils
MEDICAL EFFECTS	mucolytic
FOLK MEDICINE	meditation, encounters

American pokeweed

LATIN	Phytolacca americana (L.)
SYNONYMS	garget, pigeon-berry, pokeberry, pokeweed, scoke, Virginia poke
SPREAD	Europe, North America
PLANT PARTS	root
TEMPERATURE	200°C / 392°F
SUBSTANCES	tanning agent, saponins, acids
MEDICAL EFFECTS	anti-rheumatic, expectorant, anti-inflammatory, narcotic, pain-relieving
FOLK MEDICINE	protection, strengthening, meditation, encounters, eroticizing effect

American sweetgum

LATIN	Liquidambar styraciflua (L.)
SYNONYMS	liquidambar, American-storax, bilsted, redgum, satin-walnut, star-leaved gum, alligator-wood, sapgum
SPREAD	Europe, North America
PLANT PARTS	resin
TEMPERATURE	210°C / 410°F (max. 260°C / 500°F)
SUBSTANCES	acids
MEDICAL EFFECTS	antibacterial
FOLK MEDICINE	feeling comfortable, encounters
NOTES	False styrax (liquid amber) is often confused with the real styrax (styrax officinalis).

American witch-hazel

LATIN	Hamamelis virginiana (L.)
SYNONYMS	Witch-hazel
SPREAD	North America
PLANT PARTS	leaves, bark
TEMPERATURE	215°C / 419°F
SUBSTANCES	essential oils, flavonoids, tanning agent, acids
MEDICAL EFFECTS	antiviral, astringent, anti-inflammatory, constricting
FOLK MEDICINE	meditation, transformation, concentration, feeling comfortable, eroticizing effect

angel's trumpet

LATIN	Brugmansia (Pers.)
SYNONYMS	Daura-tree, borachero
SPREAD	Africa, Asia, Europe, North America, Oceania, South America
PLANT PARTS	herb
TEMPERATURE	220°C / 428°F
SUBSTANCES	alkaloids, glycosides
MEDICAL EFFECTS	psychoactive
FOLK MEDICINE	trance, dream, vision , eroticizing effect
NOTES	toxic

anise

LATIN	Pimpinella anisum (L.)
SYNONYMS	
SPREAD	Asia, Europe
PLANT PARTS	fruits, seeds, seeds
TEMPERATURE	190°C / 374°F
SUBSTANCES	essential oils, flavonoids, coumarins
MEDICAL EFFECTS	carminative, antispasmodic, mucolytic
FOLK MEDICINE	transformation, encounters, feeling comfortable

arolla pine

LATIN	Pinus cembra (L.)
SYNONYMS	Swiss stone pine, Austrian stone pine, Russian cedar
SPREAD	Asia, Europe
PLANT PARTS	resin, wood, needles
TEMPERATURE	230°C / 446°F
SUBSTANCES	essential oils, bittering agent, tanning agent
MEDICAL EFFECTS	anti-inflammatory, mucolytic
FOLK MEDICINE	strengthening, feeling comfortable, meditation, eroticizing effect

artichoke

LATIN	Cynara cardunculus (L.)
SYNONYMS	artichoke thistle, cardoon, cardone, cardoni, carduni, cardi
SPREAD	Africa, Asia, Europe, North America, Oceania, South America
PLANT PARTS	blossoms
TEMPERATURE	210°C / 410°F
SUBSTANCES	essential oils, bittering agent, flavonoids, tanning agent
MEDICAL EFFECTS	antioxidant
FOLK MEDICINE	cleansing, strengthening, feeling comfortable, concentration, meditation

asant

LATIN	Ferula assa-foetida (L.)
SYNONYMS	asafoetida
SPREAD	Asia
PLANT PARTS	resin
TEMPERATURE	185°C / 365°F (max. 220°C / 428°F)
SUBSTANCES	essential oils, acids
MEDICAL EFFECTS	carminative
FOLK MEDICINE	protection, feeling comfortable, transformation

ash

LATIN	Fraxinus excelsior (L.)
SYNONYMS	European ash, common ash
SPREAD	Asia, Europe, North America, Oceania
PLANT PARTS	leaves, fruits, seeds, bark
TEMPERATURE	215°C / 419°F
SUBSTANCES	essential oils, bittering agent, flavonoids, tanning agent, glycosides, coumarins, slime
MEDICAL EFFECTS	diuretic
FOLK MEDICINE	trance, dream, vision , concentration, eroticizing effect, transformation

Asian ginseng

LATIN	Panax ginseng (C.A. Mey.)
SYNONYMS	ginseng
SPREAD	Africa, Asia, Europe, North America, Oceania, South America
PLANT PARTS	root
TEMPERATURE	215°C / 419°F
SUBSTANCES	essential oils, saponins
MEDICAL EFFECTS	memory-strengthening, immuno-stimulating
FOLK MEDICINE	cleansing, encounters, concentration

Atlas cedar

LATIN	Cedrus atlantica (Manetti ex Carrière), Pinus atlantica (Endl.)
SYNONYMS	
SPREAD	Africa, Europe
PLANT PARTS	fruits, seeds, resin, ,bark
TEMPERATURE	230°C / 446°F
SUBSTANCES	essential oils, bittering agent
MEDICAL EFFECTS	antibacterial, antimycotic
FOLK MEDICINE	protection, cleansing, strengthening, eroticizing effect, transformation, feeling comfortable, concentration

autumn crocus

LATIN	Crocus sativus (L.)
SYNONYMS	saffron crocus
SPREAD	Asia, Europe
PLANT PARTS	blossoms, fibres, root
TEMPERATURE	220°C / 428°F
SUBSTANCES	essential oils
MEDICAL EFFECTS	aphrodisiac effect, appetitstimulating, calming, diuretic, antispasmodic, psychoactive
FOLK MEDICINE	encounters, trance, dream, vision , meditation, transformation, concentration

avens

LATIN	Geum urbanum (L.)
SYNONYMS	geum urbanum, herb Bennet, colewort, St. Benedict's herb
SPREAD	Africa, Asia, Europe
PLANT PARTS	root
TEMPERATURE	180°C / 356°F
SUBSTANCES	essential oils, tanning agent, glycosides
MEDICAL EFFECTS	anti-inflammatory, digestive
FOLK MEDICINE	strengthening, encounters, concentration, eroticizing effect

baloon flower

LATIN	Platycodon grandiflorus (L.)
SYNONYMS	Chinese bellflower, platycodon, radix platycodi
SPREAD	Asia, Europe, North America
PLANT PARTS	root
TEMPERATURE	230°C / 446°F
SUBSTANCES	saponins
MEDICAL EFFECTS	antiallergic, antimicrobiologic, anti-inflammatory, immuno-stimulating
FOLK MEDICINE	protection, cleansing, strengthening, eroticizing effect, feeling comfortable
NOTES	TCM-Medikament

balsam fir

LATIN	Abies balsamea (L.)
SYNONYMS	balm of Gilead, fir-balsam
SPREAD	North America
PLANT PARTS	resin, fruits, bark
TEMPERATURE	210°C / 410°F (max. 260°C / 500°F)
SUBSTANCES	essential oils
MEDICAL EFFECTS	antimicrobiologic , anti-inflammatory
FOLK MEDICINE	strengthening, encounters, concentration, feeling comfortable, meditation, eroticizing effect

balsam of Peru

LATIN	Myroxylon balsamum (Harms), Myroxylon peruiferum (L.)
SYNONYMS	balsamum peruvianum
SPREAD	South America
PLANT PARTS	resin
TEMPERATURE	220°C / 428°F (max. 280°C / 536°F)
SUBSTANCES	essential oils, acids
MEDICAL EFFECTS	antibacterial, wound-healing
FOLK MEDICINE	strengthening, transformation, feeling comfortable, encounters, concentration

baoberang

LATIN	Embelia ribes (Burm. f.)
SYNONYMS	white-flowered embelia, vidanga, false black pepper
SPREAD	Africa, Asia, Oceania, South America
PLANT PARTS	grains
TEMPERATURE	215°C / 419°F
SUBSTANCES	alkaloids, essential oils, tanning agent, acids
MEDICAL EFFECTS	anti-inflammatory, digestive
FOLK MEDICINE	cleansing, concentration, encounters, transformation, eroticizing effect
NOTES	Ayurvedic medicine

basil

LATIN	Ocimum basilicum (L.)
SYNONYMS	great basil, king of herbs, royal herb, sweet basil
SPREAD	Africa, Asia, Europe, North America, Oceania, South America
PLANT PARTS	leaves
TEMPERATURE	250°C / 482°F
SUBSTANCES	essential oils, flavonoids, tanning agent, saponins
MEDICAL EFFECTS	antimycotic, anti-inflammatory
FOLK MEDICINE	trance, dream, vision , concentration, eroticizing effect, feeling comfortable, meditation, transformation

bay laurel

LATIN	Laurus nobilis (L.)
SYNONYMS	sweet-bay, bay, true laurel, Grecian laurel
SPREAD	Asia, Europe, North America
PLANT PARTS	leaves
TEMPERATURE	245°C / 473°F
SUBSTANCES	essential oils, bittering agent
MEDICAL EFFECTS	decongestant, anti-inflammatory
FOLK MEDICINE	cleansing, strengthening, feeling comfortable, meditation, trance, dream, vision , concentration, eroticizing effect

bearberry

LATIN	Arctostaphylos uva-ursi (Spreng.)
SYNONYMS	uva-ursi, kinnikinick, pinemat manzanita, bear berry, bear-grape, creashak, hog cranberry, meal-berry, sand-berry, mountain-box
SPREAD	Europe, North America
PLANT PARTS	leaves
TEMPERATURE	220°C / 428°F
SUBSTANCES	flavonoids, tanning agent, glycosides, acids
MEDICAL EFFECTS	antibacterial, diuretic, constricting
FOLK MEDICINE	cleansing, eroticizing effect, concentration, feeling comfortable
NOTES	protected plant

bearded iris

LATIN	Iris germanica (L.)
SYNONYMS	German iris, flag, fluer-de-lis
SPREAD	Europe
PLANT PARTS	root
TEMPERATURE	200°C / 392°F
SUBSTANCES	essential oils, bittering agent, flavonoids, tanning agent, slime
MEDICAL EFFECTS	anti-inflammatory, pain-relieving
FOLK MEDICINE	encounters, trance, dream, vision , eroticizing effect

beech

LATIN	Fagus sylvatica (L.)
SYNONYMS	European beech
SPREAD	Asia, Europe, North America
PLANT PARTS	leaves
TEMPERATURE	210°C / 410°F
SUBSTANCES	fatty oil, tanning agent, saponins, acids
MEDICAL EFFECTS	anti-inflammatory
FOLK MEDICINE	transformation, eroticizing effect

belladonna

LATIN	Atropa belladonna (L.)
SYNONYMS	deadly nightshade, deadly night shade
SPREAD	Africa, Asia, Europe
PLANT PARTS	herb
TEMPERATURE	240°C / 464°F
SUBSTANCES	alkaloids, flavonoids
MEDICAL EFFECTS	psychoactive
FOLK MEDICINE	trance, dream, vision , eroticizing effect, meditation

Berber thuya

LATIN	Tetraclinis articulata (Mast.),Thuja articulata (Vahl)
SYNONYMS	sandarac tree, sictus tree, barbary thuja, arar
SPREAD	Africa, Asia
PLANT PARTS	resin
TEMPERATURE	260°C / 500°F (over 300°C / 572°F)
SUBSTANCES	essential oils
MEDICAL EFFECTS	anti-inflammatory
FOLK MEDICINE	feeling comfortable, meditation

big sagebrush

LATIN	Artemisia tridentata (Nutt.)
SYNONYMS	big sagebush, great basin sagebrush
SPREAD	North America, South America
PLANT PARTS	herb
TEMPERATURE	230°C / 446°F
SUBSTANCES	essential oils
MEDICAL EFFECTS	anti-inflammatory
FOLK MEDICINE	protection, strengthening, meditation
NOTES	The sagebrush is the national flower of the US state of Nevada.

birch

LATIN	Betula (L.)
SYNONYMS	Lockwood birch
SPREAD	Africa, Asia, Europe
PLANT PARTS	bark
TEMPERATURE	250°C / 482°F
SUBSTANCES	essential oils, bittering agent, flavonoids, tanning agent, saponins
MEDICAL EFFECTS	antimicrobiologic , antiseptic, diuretic, antispasmodic, pain-relieving, wound-healing
FOLK MEDICINE	cleansing, strengthening, concentration, feeling comfortable, transformation, meditation

Bishop's goutweed

LATIN	Aegopodium podagraria (L.)
SYNONYMS	gout-weed, ground elder, herb gerard, gout wort, snow-in-the-mountain, English masterwort, wild masterwort
SPREAD	Asia, Europe, North America
PLANT PARTS	leaves
TEMPERATURE	220°C / 428°F
SUBSTANCES	essential oils, glycosides, coumarins, acids
MEDICAL EFFECTS	anti-rheumatic
FOLK MEDICINE	protection, cleansing, transformation, eroticizing effect, meditation

bitter-grass

LATIN	Calea zacatechichi (Schltdl.), Calea ternifolia (Kunth)
SYNONYMS	Mexican calea, dream herb
SPREAD	South America
PLANT PARTS	herb
TEMPERATURE	230°C / 446°F (max.260°C / 500°F)
SUBSTANCES	alkaloids, bittering agent
MEDICAL EFFECTS	relaxing, psychoactive
FOLK MEDICINE	trance, dream, vision , eroticizing effect, concentration, transformation
NOTES	The substance is difficult to obtain on the market.

black cumin

LATIN	Nigella sativa (L.)
SYNONYMS	nigella, kalonji, black-caraway
SPREAD	Africa, Asia, Oceania, South America
PLANT PARTS	seeds
TEMPERATURE	210°C / 410°F
SUBSTANCES	essential oils, bittering agent, fatty oil, saponins, acids
MEDICAL EFFECTS	carminative, circulation-stimulating, diuretic, digestive
FOLK MEDICINE	transformation, feeling comfortable, encounters

black currant

LATIN	Ribes nigrum (L.)
SYNONYMS	European black currant, garden black currant
SPREAD	Asia, Europe
PLANT PARTS	leaves
TEMPERATURE	210°C / 410°F
SUBSTANCES	essential oils, tanning agent, glycosides, acids
MEDICAL EFFECTS	anti-inflammatory
FOLK MEDICINE	cleansing, eroticizing effect, transformation, meditation

black mustard

LATIN	Brassica nigra (W.D.J. Koch), Sinapis nigra (L.), Melanosinapis nigra (Calest.), Mutarda nigra (Bernh.), Sisymbrium nigrum (Prantl)
SYNONYMS	brown mustard, cadlock, scurvy, senvil, warlock
SPREAD	Africa, Asia, Europe, North America, Oceania, South America
PLANT PARTS	fruits, seeds, grains
TEMPERATURE	220°C / 428°F
SUBSTANCES	essential oils, glycosides, slime
MEDICAL EFFECTS	aphrodisiac effect, anti-inflammatory, digestive
FOLK MEDICINE	transformation, meditation, encounters
NOTES	May cause allergic reactions.

black pepper

LATIN	Piper nigrum (L.)
SYNONYMS	white pepper
SPREAD	Africa, Asia, Oceania, South America
PLANT PARTS	fruits, seeds, grains
TEMPERATURE	220°C / 428°F
SUBSTANCES	alkaloids, essential oils
MEDICAL EFFECTS	appetitstimulating, digestive
FOLK MEDICINE	strengthening, eroticizing effect, encounters, concentration, transformation

black raspberry

LATIN	Rubus occidentalis (L.)
SYNONYMS	European blackberry, black-cap, thimbleberry
SPREAD	Asia, Europe, North America
PLANT PARTS	leaves
TEMPERATURE	220°C / 428°F
SUBSTANCES	essential oils, flavonoids, tanning agent, acids
MEDICAL EFFECTS	dehydrating, anti-inflammatory
FOLK MEDICINE	cleansing, feeling comfortable, eroticizing effect, transformation

blackthorn

LATIN	Prunus spinosa (L.)
SYNONYMS	sloe
SPREAD	Africa, Asia, Europe, North America, Oceania
PLANT PARTS	blossoms, fruits, seeds, bark
TEMPERATURE	215°C / 419°F
SUBSTANCES	fatty oil, tanning agent, glycosides, acids
MEDICAL EFFECTS	laxative, anti-inflammatory, diuretic
FOLK MEDICINE	strengthening, eroticizing effect, encounters, transformation, concentration, feeling comfortable, meditation

blessed thistle

LATIN	Centaurea benedicta (L.), Cnicus benedictus (L.)
SYNONYMS	holy thistle, spotted thistle, St. Benedict's thistle
SPREAD	Asia, Europe
PLANT PARTS	leaves, blossoms, fruits, seeds
TEMPERATURE	205°C / 401°F
SUBSTANCES	essential oils, bittering agent, flavonoids, tanning agent, minerals, slime
MEDICAL EFFECTS	appetitstimulating, calming, pain-relieving, digestive
FOLK MEDICINE	meditation, encounters, concentration, eroticizing effect, feeling comfortable, transformation
NOTES	May cause allergic reactions.

bloodroot

LATIN	Sanguinaria canadensis (L.)
SYNONYMS	bloodwort, redroot, red-puccoon, pauson, tetterwort
SPREAD	North America
PLANT PARTS	root
TEMPERATURE	225°C / 437°F
SUBSTANCES	alkaloids
MEDICAL EFFECTS	mucolytic
FOLK MEDICINE	trance, dream, vision , concentration

bloody crane's-bill

LATIN	Geranium sanguineum (L.)
SYNONYMS	bloody geranium, blood-red geranium
SPREAD	Europe
PLANT PARTS	herb, root
TEMPERATURE	230°C / 446°F
SUBSTANCES	flavonoids, tanning agent
MEDICAL EFFECTS	dehydrating
FOLK MEDICINE	feeling comfortable, eroticizing effect

blue cohosh

LATIN	Caulophyllum thalictroides (Michx.), Leontice thalictroides (L.)
SYNONYMS	squaw root, papoose root
SPREAD	North America, South America
PLANT PARTS	root
TEMPERATURE	240°C / 464°F
SUBSTANCES	essential oils, saponins
MEDICAL EFFECTS	antispasmodic
FOLK MEDICINE	concentration, encounters

blueberry

LATIN	Vaccinium myrtillus (L.)
SYNONYMS	whortleberry, blue whortleberry, blaeberry, hurtleberry, huckleberry, winberry, fraughan, common bilberry
SPREAD	Asia, Europe, North America
PLANT PARTS	leaves
TEMPERATURE	230°C / 446°F
SUBSTANCES	tanning agent, glycosides, acids
MEDICAL EFFECTS	anti-inflammatory, wound-healing
FOLK MEDICINE	transformation, concentration, meditation, feeling comfortable, eroticizing effect

boldo

LATIN	Peumus boldus (Molina)
SYNONYMS	boldina
SPREAD	Africa, Asia, Europe, North America, Oceania, South America
PLANT PARTS	leaves
TEMPERATURE	215°C / 419°F
SUBSTANCES	alkaloids, essential oils
MEDICAL EFFECTS	bile-producing, antispasmodic
FOLK MEDICINE	eroticizing effect, meditation, trance, dream, vision , concentration

borage

LATIN	Borago officinalis (L.)
SYNONYMS	starflower, cool Tankard, tailwort, talewort
SPREAD	Asia, Europe, North America
PLANT PARTS	leaves & blossoms
TEMPERATURE	225°C / 437°F
SUBSTANCES	alkaloids, flavonoids, tanning agent, silica, saponins, acids
MEDICAL EFFECTS	antidepressant, anti-inflammatory
FOLK MEDICINE	meditation, eroticizing effect, feeling comfortable, concentration, transformation

boxwood

LATIN	Buxus sempervirens (L.)
SYNONYMS	common box, European box, Turkish boxwood
SPREAD	Africa, Asia, Europe, North America, Oceania, South America
PLANT PARTS	leaves
TEMPERATURE	220°C / 428°F
SUBSTANCES	flavonoids, tanning agent, glycosides, acids
MEDICAL EFFECTS	constricting
FOLK MEDICINE	strengthening, trance, dream, vision , feeling comfortable, concentration

breuzinho

LATIN	Protium heptaphyllum (Marchand)
SYNONYMS	Brasil resintree
SPREAD	South America
PLANT PARTS	resin
TEMPERATURE	220°C / 428°F (over 300°C / 572°F)
SUBSTANCES	essential oils
MEDICAL EFFECTS	antibacterial
FOLK MEDICINE	strengthening, transformation

buchu

LATIN	Agathosma betulina (Pillans), Hartogia betulina (P.J. Bergius)
SYNONYMS	
SPREAD	Africa
PLANT PARTS	leaves
TEMPERATURE	205°C / 401°F
SUBSTANCES	essential oils
MEDICAL EFFECTS	antibacterial, diuretic
FOLK MEDICINE	concentration

burning bush

LATIN	Dictamnus albus (L.)
SYNONYMS	dittany, fraxinella, gas plant
SPREAD	Africa, Asia, Europe
PLANT PARTS	root
TEMPERATURE	250°C / 482°F
SUBSTANCES	alkaloids, essential oils, flavonoids
MEDICAL EFFECTS	antibacterial, anti-inflammatory, anti-carcinogenic
FOLK MEDICINE	eroticizing effect, feeling comfortable, concentration, encounters

butcher's-broom

LATIN	Ruscus aculeatus (L.)
SYNONYMS	
SPREAD	Africa, Asia, Europe
PLANT PARTS	root
TEMPERATURE	210°C / 410°F
SUBSTANCES	essential oils, tanning agent, minerals, saponins
MEDICAL EFFECTS	astringent, anti-inflammatory, antipyretic, pain-relieving
FOLK MEDICINE	protection, encounters, eroticizing effect

butterbur

LATIN	Petasites hybridus (G. Gaertn., B. Mey. & Scherb.)
SYNONYMS	butterfly-dock, butter-bur, pestilence wort
SPREAD	Europe
PLANT PARTS	leaves, root
TEMPERATURE	220°C / 428°F (max. 260°C / 500°F)
SUBSTANCES	alkaloids, essential oils, slime
MEDICAL EFFECTS	antiallergic, immuno-stimulating, antispasmodic, pain-relieving
FOLK MEDICINE	strengthening, trance, dream, vision , meditation, eroticizing effect, encounters, concentration, feeling comfortable

cacao

LATIN	Theobroma cacao (L.)
SYNONYMS	cocoa tree, chocolate
SPREAD	Africa, Asia, Oceania, South America
PLANT PARTS	beans, peel
TEMPERATURE	210°C / 410°F
SUBSTANCES	alkaloids, essential oils, tanning agent
MEDICAL EFFECTS	aphrodisiac effect, blood pressure-reducing
FOLK MEDICINE	cleansing, eroticizing effect, encounters
NOTES	«dish of the gods»

California incense-cedar

LATIN	Calocedrus decurrens (Florin)
SYNONYMS	incense-cedar
SPREAD	North America
PLANT PARTS	resin, needles
TEMPERATURE	205°C / 401°F
SUBSTANCES	essential oils
MEDICAL EFFECTS	mucolytic
FOLK MEDICINE	feeling comfortable
NOTES	Difficult to find in Europe.

California poppy

LATIN	Eschscholzia californica (Cham.)
SYNONYMS	golden poppy, California sunlight, cup of gold
SPREAD	Africa, Asia, Europe, North America, Oceania, South America
PLANT PARTS	herb
TEMPERATURE	210°C / 410°F
SUBSTANCES	alkaloids, flavonoids
MEDICAL EFFECTS	psychoactive
FOLK MEDICINE	meditation, trance, dream, vision , eroticizing effect

camphor

LATIN	Cinnamomum camphora (J. Presl), Laurus camphora (L.)
SYNONYMS	camphor tree, camphorwood, camphor laurel, alcanfor
SPREAD	Africa, Asia, Oceania, South America
PLANT PARTS	crystals
TEMPERATURE	190°C / 374°F (ab 100°)
SUBSTANCES	essential oils, acids
MEDICAL EFFECTS	antiseptic, expectorant, anti-pruritic, pain-relieving, decongestant, antiepileptic, anti-inflammatory
FOLK MEDICINE	concentration, feeling comfortable, encounters, transformation, eroticizing effect, meditation
NOTES	Today camphor is mainly produced synthetically.

Canadian horseweed

LATIN	Erigeron canadensis (L.)
SYNONYMS	horseweed, Canadian fleabane, coltstail, marestail, butterweed
SPREAD	Africa, Asia, Europe, North America, Oceania, South America
PLANT PARTS	herb
TEMPERATURE	230°C / 446°F
SUBSTANCES	essential oils, tanning agent
MEDICAL EFFECTS	antibacterial, constricting
FOLK MEDICINE	protection, transformation, encounters, eroticizing effect, concentration

caraway

LATIN	Carum carvi (L.)
SYNONYMS	Persian cumin, meridian fennel
SPREAD	Africa, Asia, Europe
PLANT PARTS	leaves, fruits, seeds
TEMPERATURE	220°C / 428°F
SUBSTANCES	essential oils, fatty oil, flavonoids, tanning agent
MEDICAL EFFECTS	carminative, antispasmodic, digestive
FOLK MEDICINE	protection, feeling comfortable, encounters, transformation, concentration, eroticizing effect

cardamon

LATIN	Elettaria cardamomum (Maton)
SYNONYMS	green cardamom, true cardamom, Ceylon cardamon, Malabar cardamon
SPREAD	Africa, Asia, Oceania, South America
PLANT PARTS	fruits, seeds
TEMPERATURE	230°C / 446°F
SUBSTANCES	essential oils, glycosides
MEDICAL EFFECTS	appetitstimulating, carminative, digestive
FOLK MEDICINE	cleansing, eroticizing effect, feeling comfortable, encounters, transformation

carpetweed

LATIN	Ajuga reptans (L.), Bugula reptans (Crantz)
SYNONYMS	blue bugle, bugleherb, bugleweed, carpetweed, carpet bugleweed, ajuga
SPREAD	Africa, Asia, Europe, North America
PLANT PARTS	herb
TEMPERATURE	220°C / 428°F
SUBSTANCES	essential oils, bittering agent, glycosides, acids
MEDICAL EFFECTS	anti-inflammatory
FOLK MEDICINE	cleansing, strengthening, meditation, concentration, eroticizing effect

cat's claw

LATIN	Uncaria tomentosa (DC.)
SYNONYMS	vilcacora
SPREAD	South America
PLANT PARTS	root
TEMPERATURE	255°C / 491°F
SUBSTANCES	alkaloids, essential oils, flavonoids, acids
MEDICAL EFFECTS	anti-inflammatory, immuno-stimulating, anti-carcinogenic
FOLK MEDICINE	protection, eroticizing effect, feeling comfortable, encounters, concentration

catuaba

LATIN	Trichilia catigua (A. Juss.), Erythroxylum vaccinifolium (Mart.)
SYNONYMS	
SPREAD	South America
PLANT PARTS	wood
TEMPERATURE	230°C / 446°F
SUBSTANCES	alkaloids, essential oils
MEDICAL EFFECTS	antidepressant, invigorating
FOLK MEDICINE	feeling comfortable, encounters
NOTES	Often mixtures with Trichilia catigua, Anemopaegma arvense are sold under Catuaba.

cayenne pepper

LATIN	Capsicum annuum (L.)
SYNONYMS	bell pepper, chili pepper, chili powder, garden pepper, green pepper, mango pepper, paprika pepper,
SPREAD	Africa, Asia, Europe, North America, Oceania, South America
PLANT PARTS	fruits, seeds
TEMPERATURE	225°C / 437°F
SUBSTANCES	flavonoids, saponins
MEDICAL EFFECTS	decongestant, antibacterial, pain-relieving, digestive
FOLK MEDICINE	strengthening, eroticizing effect, feeling comfortable, transformation

celandine

LATIN	Chelidonium majus (L.)
SYNONYMS	greater celandine, tetter-wort, nipple-wort, swallow-wort, wart-weed
SPREAD	Asia, Europe, North America
PLANT PARTS	herb, root
TEMPERATURE	200°C / 392°F
SUBSTANCES	alkaloids, essential oils, bittering agent
MEDICAL EFFECTS	antibacterial, antiviral, anti-inflammatory, antispasmodic, pain-relieving
FOLK MEDICINE	protection, strengthening, eroticizing effect, encounters, meditation, transformation, concentration

celery

LATIN	Apium graveolens (L.), Celeri graveolens (Britton)
SYNONYMS	ache, celery seed, marche, march parsley, smallage, smalledge, sweet parsley, Venus's herb, wild celery
SPREAD	Africa, Asia, Europe, North America, Oceania, South America
PLANT PARTS	herb, root
TEMPERATURE	230°C / 446°F
SUBSTANCES	essential oils, flavonoids, coumarins
MEDICAL EFFECTS	diuretic, digestive
FOLK MEDICINE	strengthening, encounters, transformation, concentration, feeling comfortable

centella

LATIN	Centella asiatica (Urb.), Hydrocotyle asiatica (L.)
SYNONYMS	Asiatic pennywort, Indian pennywort, gotu kola
SPREAD	Asia
PLANT PARTS	herb
TEMPERATURE	255°C / 491°F
SUBSTANCES	essential oils, flavonoids, saponins, acids
MEDICAL EFFECTS	wound-healing
FOLK MEDICINE	feeling comfortable, concentration
NOTES	Bayer's French subsidiary SERDEX has patented five skin-care effects of the substance.

chamomile

LATIN	Matricaria chamomilla, Chamomilla rekrutita (L.)
SYNONYMS	wild chamomile, scented mayweed, false chamomile, camomile
SPREAD	Africa, Asia, Europe, North America, Oceania, South America
PLANT PARTS	blossoms
TEMPERATURE	220°C / 428°F
SUBSTANCES	essential oils, flavonoids, slime
MEDICAL EFFECTS	decongestant, carminative, antispasmodic, labor-inducing
FOLK MEDICINE	cleansing, eroticizing effect, encounters

chaste tree

LATIN	Vitex agnus-castus (L.)
SYNONYMS	chasteberry, Abraham's balm, monk's pepper, lilac chastetree
SPREAD	Asia, Europe, North America
PLANT PARTS	seeds
TEMPERATURE	220°C / 428°F
SUBSTANCES	essential oils
MEDICAL EFFECTS	hormonal
FOLK MEDICINE	trance, dream, vision , encounters

chebulic myrobalan

LATIN	Terminalia chebula (Retz.), Myrobalanus chebula (Gaertn.)
SYNONYMS	arura, black myrobalan, arjuna
SPREAD	Africa, Asia
PLANT PARTS	fruits, seeds
TEMPERATURE	210°C / 410°F
SUBSTANCES	essential oils, flavonoids, tanning agent
MEDICAL EFFECTS	dehydrating, antispasmodic
FOLK MEDICINE	feeling comfortable, encounters, transformation

chickweed

LATIN	Stellaria Media (Vill.)
SYNONYMS	common chickweed, chickenwort, craches, maruns, winterweed
SPREAD	Europe, North America
PLANT PARTS	herb
TEMPERATURE	210°C / 410°F
SUBSTANCES	flavonoids, coumarins, minerals, saponins
MEDICAL EFFECTS	pain-relieving
FOLK MEDICINE	transformation, eroticizing effect

chicory

LATIN	Cichorium intybus (L.)
SYNONYMS	barbe-de-capuchin, blue daisy, bunk, blue-sailors, coffee-weed, succory, witloof
SPREAD	Africa, Asia, Europe, North America, Oceania, South America
PLANT PARTS	herb, root
TEMPERATURE	220°C / 428°F
SUBSTANCES	essential oils, bittering agent, flavonoids, acids
MEDICAL EFFECTS	appetitstimulating, calming, digestive
FOLK MEDICINE	eroticizing effect, meditation, transformation, concentration, encounters

Chinese cinnamon

LATIN	Cinnamomum cassia (J. Presl), Laurus cassia (L.)
SYNONYMS	Chinese cassia
SPREAD	Asia
PLANT PARTS	fruits, bark, seeds
TEMPERATURE	190°C / 374°F
SUBSTANCES	essential oils, coumarins, acids
MEDICAL EFFECTS	antibacterial, antimycotic, appetitstimulating, carminative, digestive
FOLK MEDICINE	strengthening, feeling comfortable, encounters, transformation

Chinese foxglove

LATIN	Rehmannia glutinosa (Libosch. ex Fisch. & C.A. Mey.)
SYNONYMS	di huang
SPREAD	Asia
PLANT PARTS	root
TEMPERATURE	220°C / 428°F
SUBSTANCES	glycosides
MEDICAL EFFECTS	antibacterial, anti-inflammatory, diuretic
FOLK MEDICINE	eroticizing effect
NOTES	Use in traditional Chinese medicine.

Chinese rhubarb

LATIN	Rheum palmatum (L.)
SYNONYMS	ornamental rhubarb, Turkish rhubarb, Indian rhubarb, Russian rhubarb
SPREAD	Asia
PLANT PARTS	root
TEMPERATURE	220°C / 428°F
SUBSTANCES	anthranoids, flavonoids, tanning agent, acids
MEDICAL EFFECTS	laxative, appetitstimulating
FOLK MEDICINE	feeling comfortable, eroticizing effect, concentration

Chinese witch hazel

LATIN	Hamamelis mollis (Oliv.)
SYNONYMS	
SPREAD	Asia
PLANT PARTS	leaves, blossoms
TEMPERATURE	210°C / 410°F
SUBSTANCES	essential oils, flavonoids, tanning agent, acids
MEDICAL EFFECTS	antiviral, astringent, anti-inflammatory, constricting
FOLK MEDICINE	meditation, concentration, encounters, eroticizing effect, feeling comfortable, transformation

christmas rose

LATIN	Helleborus niger (L.)
SYNONYMS	black hellebore
SPREAD	Asia, Europe
PLANT PARTS	root
TEMPERATURE	220°C / 428°F
SUBSTANCES	anthranoids, glycosides, saponins
MEDICAL EFFECTS	laxative, paralyzing
FOLK MEDICINE	protection, trance, dream, vision , feeling comfortable, meditation
NOTES	highly toxic

cinnamon

LATIN	Canella alba (Murray), Canella winterana (Gaertn.)
SYNONYMS	cinnamon bark, wild cinnamon, white cinnamon, canella
SPREAD	Africa, Asia, Oceania, South America
PLANT PARTS	bark
TEMPERATURE	210°C / 410°F
SUBSTANCES	essential oils, tanning agent, slime
MEDICAL EFFECTS	constricting
FOLK MEDICINE	strengthening, trance, dream, vision , feeling comfortable, concentration

cinnamon

LATIN	Cinnamomum verum (J. Presl)
SYNONYMS	Ceylon cinnamon tree, true cinnamon
SPREAD	Africa, Asia
PLANT PARTS	blossoms, bark
TEMPERATURE	240°C / 464°F
SUBSTANCES	essential oils, tanning agent, slime
MEDICAL EFFECTS	antimicrobiologic , labor-inducing
FOLK MEDICINE	strengthening, feeling comfortable, encounters

citron

LATIN	Citrus medica (L.), Aurantium medicum (M. Gómez)
SYNONYMS	lemon, citrus
SPREAD	Africa, Asia, Oceania, South America
PLANT PARTS	fruits, seeds, peel
TEMPERATURE	205°C / 401°F
SUBSTANCES	essential oils, flavonoids, acids
MEDICAL EFFECTS	antibacterial
FOLK MEDICINE	cleansing, eroticizing effect
NOTES	One of the 4 holy Jewish plants (myrtle, date palm, willow, lemon).

clary sage

LATIN	Salvia sclarea (L.)
SYNONYMS	European sage
SPREAD	Asia, Europe
PLANT PARTS	herb
TEMPERATURE	225°C / 437°F
SUBSTANCES	essential oils
MEDICAL EFFECTS	antispasmodic, digestive
FOLK MEDICINE	encounters, meditation, transformation

clovetree

LATIN	Syzygium aromaticum (Merr. & L.M. Perry)
SYNONYMS	cloves
SPREAD	Asia
PLANT PARTS	blossoms
TEMPERATURE	200°C / 392°F
SUBSTANCES	essential oils, flavonoids, tanning agent, acids
MEDICAL EFFECTS	antibacterial, pain-relieving
FOLK MEDICINE	strengthening, encounters, feeling comfortable, meditation

coco-grass

LATIN	Cyperus rotundus (L.)
SYNONYMS	Java grass, coco sedge, coco-grass, nut grass, purple nut sedge, red nut sedge
SPREAD	Africa, Asia, Europe, North America, Oceania, South America
PLANT PARTS	root
TEMPERATURE	240°C / 464°F
SUBSTANCES	alkaloids, essential oils, flavonoids, glycosides
MEDICAL EFFECTS	antibacterial, diuretic
FOLK MEDICINE	cleansing, eroticizing effect, concentration, encounters

coffee

LATIN	Coffea arabica (L.), Coffea canephora (Pierre ex A. Froehner)
SYNONYMS	coffee shrub of Arabia, mountain coffee, arabica coffee, wild robusta coffee
SPREAD	Africa, Asia, Oceania, South America
PLANT PARTS	beans, fruits, seeds
TEMPERATURE	205°C / 401°F
SUBSTANCES	alkaloids, essential oils, acids
MEDICAL EFFECTS	stoffwechselstimulating
FOLK MEDICINE	concentration

coltsfoot

LATIN	Tussilago farfara (L.)
SYNONYMS	
SPREAD	Asia, Europe, North America
PLANT PARTS	leaves, blossoms
TEMPERATURE	210°C / 410°F
SUBSTANCES	alkaloids, essential oils, bittering agent, tanning agent, minerals, saponins, acids, slime
MEDICAL EFFECTS	mucolytic
FOLK MEDICINE	trance, dream, vision , concentration, meditation, encounters

common barberry

LATIN	Berberis vulgaris (L.)
SYNONYMS	European barberry, simply barberry, piprage
SPREAD	Asia, Europe
PLANT PARTS	rootbark
TEMPERATURE	235°C / 455°F
SUBSTANCES	alkaloids, tanning agent
MEDICAL EFFECTS	lowering bloog sugar levels
FOLK MEDICINE	protection, feeling comfortable

common boneset

LATIN	Eupatorium perfoliatum (L.)
SYNONYMS	feverweed, purple boneset, sweating-plant, thoroughwort
SPREAD	Europe, North America
PLANT PARTS	herb
TEMPERATURE	220°C / 428°F
SUBSTANCES	alkaloids, essential oils, flavonoids, tanning agent, glycosides, saponins
MEDICAL EFFECTS	laxative, expectorant, diuretic, immuno-stimulating
FOLK MEDICINE	cleansing, eroticizing effect, encounters, feeling comfortable, transformation, concentration, meditation

common broom

LATIN	Sarothamnus scoparius (W.D.J. Koch)
SYNONYMS	Scotch broom, English broom
SPREAD	Europe
PLANT PARTS	leaves, blossoms
TEMPERATURE	220°C / 428°F
SUBSTANCES	essential oils, flavonoids
MEDICAL EFFECTS	blood pressure-regulating
FOLK MEDICINE	concentration, encounters, eroticizing effect

common bugloss

LATIN	Anchusa officinalis (Gouan)
SYNONYMS	alkanet
SPREAD	Europe, North America
PLANT PARTS	herb, root
TEMPERATURE	210°C / 410°F
SUBSTANCES	alkaloids, flavonoids, tanning agent, silica, saponins, slime
MEDICAL EFFECTS	dehydrating, diuretic, mucolytic
FOLK MEDICINE	eroticizing effect, concentration, transformation, encounters, feeling comfortable

common centaury

LATIN	Centaurium erythraea (Rafn)
SYNONYMS	European centaury
SPREAD	Europe
PLANT PARTS	herb
TEMPERATURE	220°C / 428°F
SUBSTANCES	bittering agent, flavonoids, acids
MEDICAL EFFECTS	appetitstimulating
FOLK MEDICINE	transformation, eroticizing effect

common comfrey

LATIN	Symphytum officinale (L.)
SYNONYMS	
SPREAD	Africa, Asia, Europe
PLANT PARTS	leaves, root
TEMPERATURE	215°C / 419°F
SUBSTANCES	alkaloids, essential oils, flavonoids, tanning agent, silica, slime
MEDICAL EFFECTS	decongestant, anti-inflammatory, pain-relieving
FOLK MEDICINE	cleansing, meditation, eroticizing effect, concentration, feeling comfortable, encounters, transformation

common dandelion

LATIN	Taraxacum officinale (F.H. Wigg.)
SYNONYMS	dandelion
SPREAD	Africa, Asia, Europe, North America, Oceania, South America
PLANT PARTS	herb, root
TEMPERATURE	240°C / 464°F
SUBSTANCES	bittering agent, glycosides, minerals
MEDICAL EFFECTS	appetitstimulating, diuretic, anti-carcinogenic , digestive
FOLK MEDICINE	transformation, concentration, meditation, eroticizing effect, feeling comfortable, encounters

common evening primrose

LATIN	Oenothera biennis (L.)
SYNONYMS	evening star, sun drop, fever-plant, field-primrose, German rampion, tree-primrose, yellow evening-primrose
SPREAD	Asia, Europe, North America
PLANT PARTS	leaves
TEMPERATURE	195°C / 383°F
SUBSTANCES	tanning agent, acids, slime
MEDICAL EFFECTS	anti-inflammatory
FOLK MEDICINE	transformation, eroticizing effect, encounters

common gypsyweed

LATIN	Veronica officinalis (L.)
SYNONYMS	common speedwell, heath speedwell, Paul's betony
SPREAD	Asia, Europe
PLANT PARTS	herb
TEMPERATURE	225°C / 437°F
SUBSTANCES	essential oils, bittering agent, tanning agent, saponins, acids
MEDICAL EFFECTS	anti-rheumatic, cough suppressant
FOLK MEDICINE	cleansing, strengthening, concentration, meditation, eroticizing effect, transformation

common holly

LATIN	Ilex aquifolium (L.)
SYNONYMS	European holly, English holly, christmas holly
SPREAD	Africa, Asia, Europe
PLANT PARTS	leaves
TEMPERATURE	245°C / 473°F
SUBSTANCES	bittering agent, tanning agent, glycosides
MEDICAL EFFECTS	antipyretic, diuretic
FOLK MEDICINE	eroticizing effect, concentration
NOTES	Fruits are toxic.

common hollyhock

LATIN	Alcea rosea (L.), Althaea rosea (Cav.)
SYNONYMS	
SPREAD	Europe
PLANT PARTS	leaves, blossoms, root
TEMPERATURE	240°C / 464°F
SUBSTANCES	tanning agent, slime
MEDICAL EFFECTS	cough suppressant, constricting
FOLK MEDICINE	protection, encounters, concentration

common hop

LATIN	Humulus lupulus (L.)
SYNONYMS	bine, European hop
SPREAD	Africa, Asia, Europe, North America, Oceania, South America
PLANT PARTS	blossoms
TEMPERATURE	215°C / 419°F
SUBSTANCES	essential oils, bittering agent, acids
MEDICAL EFFECTS	antibacterial, calming, soporific
FOLK MEDICINE	trance, dream, vision , encounters, meditation

common houseleek

LATIN	Sempervivum tectorum (L.)
SYNONYMS	conchita, rosa verde
SPREAD	Asia, Europe
PLANT PARTS	leaves
TEMPERATURE	240°C / 464°F
SUBSTANCES	tanning agent, acids, slime
MEDICAL EFFECTS	antipyretic, antispasmodic, pain-relieving
FOLK MEDICINE	eroticizing effect, encounters, meditation, feeling comfortable

common juniper

LATIN	Juniperus communis (L.)
SYNONYMS	mountain juniper, savin, magician's cypress, devil's tree
SPREAD	Asia, Europe, North America
PLANT PARTS	berries, leaves, fruits, seeds, wood
TEMPERATURE	220°C / 428°F
SUBSTANCES	essential oils, bittering agent, tanning agent, acids
MEDICAL EFFECTS	decongestant, antipyretic, diuretic
FOLK MEDICINE	cleansing, strengthening, eroticizing effect, concentration
NOTES	Was considered a universal remedy in folk medicine.

common licorice

LATIN	Glycyrrhiza glabra (L.)
SYNONYMS	Licorice-root, wild licorice
SPREAD	Asia, Europe
PLANT PARTS	root
TEMPERATURE	225°C / 437°F
SUBSTANCES	flavonoids, coumarins, saponins, acids
MEDICAL EFFECTS	antibacterial, antimicrobiologic , anti-inflammatory, antispasmodic, mucolytic
FOLK MEDICINE	eroticizing effect, encounters, meditation

common motherwort

LATIN	Leonurus cardiaca (L.)
SYNONYMS	throw-wort, lion's ear, lion's tail
SPREAD	Asia, Europe, North America
PLANT PARTS	herb
TEMPERATURE	210°C / 410°F
SUBSTANCES	essential oils
MEDICAL EFFECTS	calming
FOLK MEDICINE	eroticizing effect, feeling comfortable, transformation

common poppy

LATIN	Papaver rhoeas (L.)
SYNONYMS	corn poppy, corn rose, field poppy, Flanders poppy, red poppy, red weed
SPREAD	Africa, Asia, Europe
PLANT PARTS	blossoms
TEMPERATURE	205°C / 401°F
SUBSTANCES	alkaloids, glycosides, slime
MEDICAL EFFECTS	calming
FOLK MEDICINE	protection, meditation, eroticizing effect

common ragwort

LATIN	Jacobaea vulgaris (Gaertn.), Senecio jacobaea (L.)
SYNONYMS	tansy ragwort, stinking willie, benweed, St. James-wort, stinking nanny, staggerwort, dog standard, cankerwort, stammerwort, mare's fart, cushag
SPREAD	Africa, Asia, Europe, North America, Oceania, South America
PLANT PARTS	herb
TEMPERATURE	220°C / 428°F
SUBSTANCES	essential oils, flavonoids, tanning agent, silica
MEDICAL EFFECTS	decongestant, anti-inflammatory
FOLK MEDICINE	protection, meditation, transformation
NOTES	Toxic even when dried.

common rue

LATIN	Ruta graveolens (L.)
SYNONYMS	rue, herb-of-grace
SPREAD	Africa, Europe
PLANT PARTS	herb
TEMPERATURE	230°C / 446°F
SUBSTANCES	alkaloids,essential oils,bittering agent,glycosides,coumarins,acids
MEDICAL EFFECTS	antibacterial,antispasmodic,pain-relieving,labor-inducing
FOLK MEDICINE	protection, strengthening, eroticizing effect, encounters, transformation, meditation
NOTES	The plant is phototoxic, i.e. it can cause skin irritation when touched and exposed to sunlight.

common sage

LATIN	Salvia officinalis (L.)
SYNONYMS	garden sage
SPREAD	Europe
PLANT PARTS	leaves
TEMPERATURE	210°C / 410°F
SUBSTANCES	essential oils, bittering agent, flavonoids, tanning agent, acids
MEDICAL EFFECTS	antibacterial, antiviral, diuretic, antispasmodic
FOLK MEDICINE	cleansing, strengthening, eroticizing effect, concentration, meditation

common tansy

LATIN	Tanacetum vulgare (L.)
SYNONYMS	bitter buttons, cow bitter, golden buttons
SPREAD	Africa, Asia, Europe, North America, Oceania, South America
PLANT PARTS	herb
TEMPERATURE	225°C / 437°F
SUBSTANCES	anthranoids, essential oils, bittering agent, tanning agent, glycosides
MEDICAL EFFECTS	laxative, antiviral
FOLK MEDICINE	strengthening, eroticizing effect, meditation

common thorn apple

LATIN	Datura stramonium (L.)
SYNONYMS	jimsonweed, devil's snare, moon flower, toloache. hell's bells, devil's trumpet, devil's weed, Jamestown weed, stinkweed, locoweed, pricklyburr, devil's cucumber
SPREAD	Africa, Asia, Europe, North America, Oceania, South America
PLANT PARTS	leaves, fruits, seeds
TEMPERATURE	240°C / 464°F
SUBSTANCES	alkaloids, flavonoids, coumarins
MEDICAL EFFECTS	antispasmodic, psychoactive, pain-relieving
FOLK MEDICINE	protection, trance, dream, vision , eroticizing effect, concentration, transformation, feeling comfortable, meditation
NOTES	toxic

common yew

LATIN	Taxus baccata (L.)
SYNONYMS	English yew, European yew
SPREAD	Africa, Asia, Europe
PLANT PARTS	needles
TEMPERATURE	220°C / 428°F
SUBSTANCES	essential oils, glycosides
MEDICAL EFFECTS	anti-carcinogenic
FOLK MEDICINE	protection, transformation

condorvine

LATIN	Marsdenia cundurango (Rchb. f.)
SYNONYMS	cundurango
SPREAD	South America
PLANT PARTS	bark
TEMPERATURE	215°C / 419°F
SUBSTANCES	bittering agent, glycosides
MEDICAL EFFECTS	appetitstimulating
FOLK MEDICINE	transformation, concentration

copaiba balsam

LATIN	Copaifera officinalis (L.), Copaiva officinalis (Jacq.)
SYNONYMS	copal-bearer, copaiba-bearer
SPREAD	Africa, Asia, Oceania, South America
PLANT PARTS	resin
TEMPERATURE	200°C / 392°F (max. 260°C / 500°F)
SUBSTANCES	essential oils, acids
MEDICAL EFFECTS	antibacterial, antimycotic, anti-inflammatory
FOLK MEDICINE	protection, eroticizing effect, meditation, transformation, encounters, feeling comfortable
NOTES	May cause allergic reactions.

copal black

LATIN	Bursera glabrifolia (Engl.), Protium copal (Engl.)
SYNONYMS	
SPREAD	South America
PLANT PARTS	resin
TEMPERATURE	260°C / 500°F (over 300°C / 572°F)
SUBSTANCES	essential oils, bittering agent, acids
MEDICAL EFFECTS	antiseptic
FOLK MEDICINE	eroticizing effect, feeling comfortable, concentration, trance, dream, vision , transformation

copal white

LATIN	Bursera bipinnata (Engl.), Amyris bipinnata (DC.)
SYNONYMS	
SPREAD	South America
PLANT PARTS	resin
TEMPERATURE	240°C / 464°F (over 300°C / 572°F)
SUBSTANCES	essential oils, bittering agent, acids
MEDICAL EFFECTS	antiseptic
FOLK MEDICINE	eroticizing effect, feeling comfortable, concentration, trance, dream, vision , transformation

coriander

LATIN	Coriandrum sativum (L.)
SYNONYMS	cilantro, Chinese parsley
SPREAD	Africa, Asia, Europe, North America, Oceania, South America
PLANT PARTS	fruits, seeds
TEMPERATURE	215°C / 419°F
SUBSTANCES	essential oils, tanning agent, coumarins, acids
MEDICAL EFFECTS	appetitstimulating, antispasmodic, digestive
FOLK MEDICINE	feeling comfortable, encounters, transformation

corn silk

LATIN	Zea mays (L.)
SYNONYMS	maize
SPREAD	Africa, Asia, Europe, North America, Oceania, South America
PLANT PARTS	fibres
TEMPERATURE	210°C / 410°F
SUBSTANCES	essential oils, fatty oil, acids
MEDICAL EFFECTS	diuretic
FOLK MEDICINE	encounters, eroticizing effect

cornflower

LATIN	Centaurea cyanus (L.)
SYNONYMS	Bachelor's-button, bluebottle
SPREAD	Asia, Europe, North America
PLANT PARTS	herb, plant
TEMPERATURE	225°C / 437°F
SUBSTANCES	bittering agent, flavonoids, tanning agent, glycosides, slime
MEDICAL EFFECTS	anti-inflammatory
FOLK MEDICINE	protection, concentration, transformation, meditation, eroticizing effect

costmary

LATIN	Tanacetum balsamita (L.), Balsamita vulgaris (Willd.)
SYNONYMS	alecost, balsam herb, bible leaf, mint geranium
SPREAD	Asia, Europe
PLANT PARTS	leaves
TEMPERATURE	225°C / 437°F
SUBSTANCES	essential oils, acids
MEDICAL EFFECTS	antiseptic, diuretic, antispasmodic
FOLK MEDICINE	transformation, concentration, meditation, eroticizing effect

costus

LATIN	Saussurea costus (Lipsch.), Aucklandia costus (Falc.)
SYNONYMS	kuth
SPREAD	Asia
PLANT PARTS	root
TEMPERATURE	190°C / 374°F
SUBSTANCES	essential oils
MEDICAL EFFECTS	immuno-stimulating
FOLK MEDICINE	eroticizing effect, encounters

cowslip

LATIN	Primula veris (L.)
SYNONYMS	common cowslip, cowslip primrose
SPREAD	Asia, Europe
PLANT PARTS	blossoms, root
TEMPERATURE	210°C / 410°F
SUBSTANCES	essential oils, flavonoids, tanning agent, glycosides, silica, saponins
MEDICAL EFFECTS	dehydrating, mucolytic
FOLK MEDICINE	strengthening, encounters, eroticizing effect, meditation
NOTES	protected plant

curry tree

LATIN	Bergera koenigii (L.), Chalcas koenigii (Kurz), Murraya koenigii (Spreng.)
SYNONYMS	
SPREAD	Asia
PLANT PARTS	leaves, fruits, bark, root
TEMPERATURE	220°C / 428°F
SUBSTANCES	essential oils
MEDICAL EFFECTS	antimicrobiologic
FOLK MEDICINE	cleansing, strengthening, concentration, encounters, feeling comfortable, meditation
NOTES	Ayurvedic medicine

damiana

LATIN	Turnera diffusa (Willd.)
SYNONYMS	oreganillo, Mexican holly
SPREAD	North America, South America
PLANT PARTS	leaves
TEMPERATURE	240°C / 464°F
SUBSTANCES	essential oils, bittering agent, tanning agent
MEDICAL EFFECTS	calming, antispasmodic, psychoactive
FOLK MEDICINE	eroticizing effect, encounters, trance, dream, vision , concentration

denseflower mullein

LATIN	Verbascum densiflorum (Bertol.)
SYNONYMS	dense-flowered mullein
SPREAD	Europe
PLANT PARTS	leaves, blossoms, fruits, seeds
TEMPERATURE	220°C / 428°F
SUBSTANCES	essential oils, flavonoids, coumarins, saponins, slime
MEDICAL EFFECTS	anti-inflammatory
FOLK MEDICINE	strengthening, trance, dream, vision , eroticizing effect, encounters, transformation, feeling comfortable, meditation

deodar cedar

LATIN	Cedrus deodara (G. Don), Pinus deodara (Roxb. ex D. Don)
SYNONYMS	Himalayan cedar, deodar, devdar, devadar, devadaru
SPREAD	Asia, Europe, North America
PLANT PARTS	resin
TEMPERATURE	230°C / 446°F (over 300°C / 572°F)
SUBSTANCES	essential oils
MEDICAL EFFECTS	antimycotic, constricting
FOLK MEDICINE	eroticizing effect, encounters

desert parsley

LATIN	Lomatium dissectum (Mathias & Constance)
SYNONYMS	fernleaf biscuitroot
SPREAD	North America
PLANT PARTS	root
TEMPERATURE	240°C / 464°F
SUBSTANCES	essential oils, tanning agent, glycosides, coumarins, saponins, acids
MEDICAL EFFECTS	antibacterial, antiviral
FOLK MEDICINE	concentration, encounters, feeling comfortable, meditation, eroticizing effect

diesel tree

LATIN	Copaifera langsdorffii (Desf.), Copaiba langsdorfii (Kuntze)
SYNONYMS	
SPREAD	Africa
PLANT PARTS	resin
TEMPERATURE	230°C / 446°F (over 300°C / 572°F)
SUBSTANCES	essential oils, bittering agent, acids
MEDICAL EFFECTS	antiseptic
FOLK MEDICINE	eroticizing effect, feeling comfortable, concentration, trance, dream, vision , transformation

dill

LATIN	Anethum graveolens (L.)
SYNONYMS	Dill
SPREAD	Asia, Europe
PLANT PARTS	fruits, seeds, herb
TEMPERATURE	220°C / 428°F
SUBSTANCES	anthranoids, essential oils, coumarins, minerals, acids
MEDICAL EFFECTS	laxative, antispasmodic
FOLK MEDICINE	eroticizing effect, concentration, transformation, meditation, feeling comfortable

dog rose

LATIN	Rosa canina (L.)
SYNONYMS	dog-brier
SPREAD	Africa, Asia, Europe, North America
PLANT PARTS	blossoms, fruits, seeds
TEMPERATURE	200°C / 392°F
SUBSTANCES	essential oils, fatty oil, tanning agent, saponins, acids
MEDICAL EFFECTS	immuno-stimulating
FOLK MEDICINE	eroticizing effect, encounters, meditation, trance, dream, vision , transformation

dog's mercury

LATIN	Mercurialis perennis (L.)
SYNONYMS	
SPREAD	Africa, Asia, Europe
PLANT PARTS	leaves
TEMPERATURE	215°C / 419°F
SUBSTANCES	saponins
MEDICAL EFFECTS	laxative
FOLK MEDICINE	concentration

Douglas' sagewort

LATIN	Artemisia douglasiana (Besser)
SYNONYMS	California mugwort, Douglas's mugwort, dream plant, Northwest mugwort
SPREAD	North America, South America
PLANT PARTS	herb
TEMPERATURE	260°C / 500°F
SUBSTANCES	essential oils
MEDICAL EFFECTS	germicidal
FOLK MEDICINE	concentration

dragon's blood

LATIN	Dracaena cinnabari (Balf. f.), Daemonorops draco (Blume)
SYNONYMS	Socotra dragon tree, Sumatra dragon´s blood
SPREAD	Africa, Asia
PLANT PARTS	resin
TEMPERATURE	250°C / 482°F (max. 280°C / 536°F)
SUBSTANCES	essential oils, acids
MEDICAL EFFECTS	antiseptic
FOLK MEDICINE	protection, strengthening, feeling comfortable, concentration

drug snowbell

LATIN	Styrax officinalis (L.)
SYNONYMS	Friar's balsam, storax
SPREAD	Asia, Europe, North America
PLANT PARTS	resin, bark
TEMPERATURE	265°C / 509°F (over 300°C / 572°F)
SUBSTANCES	essential oils, acids
MEDICAL EFFECTS	antiseptic, calming, mucolytic
FOLK MEDICINE	feeling comfortable, encounters, transformation, concentration

dwarf everlasting

LATIN	Helichrysum arenarium (Moench)
SYNONYMS	immortelle
SPREAD	Asia, Europe
PLANT PARTS	herb
TEMPERATURE	225°C / 437°F
SUBSTANCES	essential oils, bittering agent, flavonoids, glycosides, coumarins, acids
MEDICAL EFFECTS	diuretic, cough suppressant
FOLK MEDICINE	strengthening, meditation, transformation, encounters

dwarf thistle

LATIN	Carlina acaulis (L.)
SYNONYMS	dwarf carline thistle, silver thistle
SPREAD	Europe
PLANT PARTS	blossoms, root
TEMPERATURE	200°C / 392°F
SUBSTANCES	essential oils, bittering agent, flavonoids, tanning agent
MEDICAL EFFECTS	anti-inflammatory
FOLK MEDICINE	encounters, meditation
NOTES	Protected plant that can cause allergic reactions.

eastern juniper

LATIN	Juniperus polycarpos (K.Koch), Juniperus excelsa (M. Bieb.)
SYNONYMS	greek juniper, Pashtun juniper
SPREAD	Asia
PLANT PARTS	leaves
TEMPERATURE	220°C / 428°F
SUBSTANCES	essential oils, bittering agent, tanning agent, acids
MEDICAL EFFECTS	decongestant, antipyretic, diuretic
FOLK MEDICINE	strengthening, concentration, eroticizing effect

eastern teaberry

LATIN	Gaultheria procumbens (L.)
SYNONYMS	American wintergreen, boxberry, checkerberry, mountain-tea, teaberry
SPREAD	North America
PLANT PARTS	leaves
TEMPERATURE	220°C / 428°F
SUBSTANCES	essential oils, tanning agent
MEDICAL EFFECTS	anti-inflammatory, pain-relieving
FOLK MEDICINE	cleansing, eroticizing effect, feeling comfortable, transformation, encounters

elderberry

LATIN	Sambucus nigra (L.)
SYNONYMS	elder, black elder, European elder, European black elderberry
SPREAD	Asia, Europe, North America
PLANT PARTS	blossoms, fruits, seeds, wood, bark
TEMPERATURE	210°C / 410°F
SUBSTANCES	essential oils, flavonoids, tanning agent, acids, slime
MEDICAL EFFECTS	immuno-stimulating
FOLK MEDICINE	strengthening, meditation, transformation, eroticizing effect

elecampane

LATIN	Inula helenium (L.)
SYNONYMS	horse-heal, elf-dock, elf-wort, horse-elder, scab-wort, yellow starwort
SPREAD	Asia, Europe
PLANT PARTS	root
TEMPERATURE	180°C / 356°F
SUBSTANCES	essential oils, bittering agent, acids
MEDICAL EFFECTS	expectorant, disinfectant
FOLK MEDICINE	protection, cleansing, eroticizing effect, meditation

elemi

LATIN	Canarium luzonicum (A. Gray
SYNONYMS	
SPREAD	Asia
PLANT PARTS	resin
TEMPERATURE	250°C / 482°F (over 300°C / 572°F)
SUBSTANCES	essential oils, acids
MEDICAL EFFECTS	wound-healing
FOLK MEDICINE	cleansing, strengthening, concentration, feeling comfortable
NOTES	fresh, sticky resin

elemi frankincense

LATIN	Boswellia frereana (Birdw.)
SYNONYMS	dhidin, maydi, king of all frankincense, yigaar, coptic frankincense
SPREAD	Africa
PLANT PARTS	resin
TEMPERATURE	230°C / 446°F (over 300°C / 572°F)
SUBSTANCES	essential oils, acids
MEDICAL EFFECTS	wound-healing
FOLK MEDICINE	cleansing, strengthening, concentration, feeling comfortable

elm

LATIN	Ulmus (L.)
SYNONYMS	
SPREAD	Asia, Europe, North America
PLANT PARTS	leaves
TEMPERATURE	225°C / 437°F
SUBSTANCES	bittering agent, tanning agent, slime
MEDICAL EFFECTS	anti-inflammatory, diuretic, wound-healing, constricting
FOLK MEDICINE	concentration, transformation, encounters

English daisy

LATIN	Bellis perennis (L.)
SYNONYMS	common daisy, English daisy, European daisy, bruisewort, woundwort, lawn daisy
SPREAD	Asia, Europe, North America, Oceania
PLANT PARTS	leaves
TEMPERATURE	230°C / 446°F
SUBSTANCES	essential oils, bittering agent, flavonoids, tanning agent, saponins, slime
MEDICAL EFFECTS	antimicrobiologic , stoffwechselstimulating
FOLK MEDICINE	strengthening, concentration, encounters, meditation, eroticizing effect

English ivy

LATIN	Hedera helix (L.)
SYNONYMS	European ivy
SPREAD	Asia, Europe, North America, Oceania
PLANT PARTS	leaves, fruits
TEMPERATURE	200°C / 392°F
SUBSTANCES	essential oils, flavonoids, saponins
MEDICAL EFFECTS	antispasmodic, mucolytic
FOLK MEDICINE	concentration, encounters, meditation, feeling comfortable, eroticizing effect
NOTES	All parts of the plant are toxic.

English lavender

LATIN	Lavandula angustifolia (Mill.)
SYNONYMS	true lavender, common lavender, narrow-leaved lavender
SPREAD	Europe
PLANT PARTS	blossoms
TEMPERATURE	260°C / 500°F
SUBSTANCES	essential oils, tanning agent, coumarins
MEDICAL EFFECTS	calming
FOLK MEDICINE	cleansing, strengthening, eroticizing effect, feeling comfortable, meditation, trance, dream, vision , encounters

erect cinquefoil

LATIN	Potentilla erecta (L.)
SYNONYMS	septfoil, tormentil
SPREAD	Asia, Europe, North America
PLANT PARTS	leaves, root
TEMPERATURE	220°C / 428°F
SUBSTANCES	essential oils, tanning agent, glycosides, acids
MEDICAL EFFECTS	antibacterial, antiviral, dehydrating, anti-inflammatory
FOLK MEDICINE	concentration, meditation, encounters, feeling comfortable, eroticizing effect, transformation

eucalyptus

LATIN	Eucalyptus globulus (Labill.)
SYNONYMS	Tasmanian bluegum, southern blue-gum, bluegum eucalyptus
SPREAD	Africa, Asia, Europe, North America, Oceania, South America
PLANT PARTS	leaves
TEMPERATURE	235°C / 455°F
SUBSTANCES	essential oils, flavonoids, acids
MEDICAL EFFECTS	anti-inflammatory, antipyretic
FOLK MEDICINE	strengthening, eroticizing effect, feeling comfortable

European alder

LATIN	Alnus glutinosa (L.)
SYNONYMS	common alder, black alder
SPREAD	Africa, Asia, Europe, North America
PLANT PARTS	leaves, fruits, seeds
TEMPERATURE	230°C / 446°F
SUBSTANCES	flavonoids, tanning agent
MEDICAL EFFECTS	anti-inflammatory
FOLK MEDICINE	cleansing, strengthening, feeling comfortable, encounters, transformation

European aspen

LATIN	Populus tremula (L.)
SYNONYMS	common aspen, Eurasian aspen, quaking aspen
SPREAD	Africa, Asia, Europe
PLANT PARTS	leaves, resin
TEMPERATURE	210°C / 410°F
SUBSTANCES	essential oils, flavonoids, tanning agent, glycosides
MEDICAL EFFECTS	disinfectant, pain-relieving, wound-healing
FOLK MEDICINE	cleansing, feeling comfortable, encounters, concentration, meditation

European columbine

LATIN	Aquilegia vulgaris (L.)
SYNONYMS	garden columbine, garden crowfoot, European crowfoot, Granny's nightcap, Granny's bonnet
SPREAD	Africa, Asia, Europe
PLANT PARTS	herb
TEMPERATURE	220°C / 428°F
SUBSTANCES	alkaloids, essential oils, flavonoids, glycosides
MEDICAL EFFECTS	nervine
FOLK MEDICINE	eroticizing effect, transformation
NOTES	protected plant, slightly poisonous

European goldenrod

LATIN	Solidago virgaurea (L.)
SYNONYMS	woundwort, goldenrod
SPREAD	Africa, Asia, Europe, North America, Oceania, South America
PLANT PARTS	herb
TEMPERATURE	225°C / 437°F
SUBSTANCES	essential oils, bittering agent, flavonoids, tanning agent, saponins
MEDICAL EFFECTS	anti-inflammatory, antispasmodic, pain-relieving
FOLK MEDICINE	protection, meditation, transformation, concentration, eroticizing effect

European grape

LATIN	Vitis vinifera (L.)
SYNONYMS	wine grape
SPREAD	Africa, Asia, Europe, North America, Oceania, South America
PLANT PARTS	leaves, blossoms
TEMPERATURE	190°C / 374°F
SUBSTANCES	tanning agent, minerals, acids
MEDICAL EFFECTS	constricting
FOLK MEDICINE	cleansing, concentration, encounters, feeling comfortable

European larch

LATIN	Larix decidua (Mill.)
SYNONYMS	creosote bush
SPREAD	Europe
PLANT PARTS	leaves, resin, bark
TEMPERATURE	250°C / 482°F (over 300°C / 572°F)
SUBSTANCES	essential oils, bittering agent, acids
MEDICAL EFFECTS	antiseptic, expectorant, circulation-stimulating
FOLK MEDICINE	cleansing, strengthening, transformation, feeling comfortable, meditation, concentration, encounters

fennel

LATIN	Foeniculum vulgare (Mill.)
SYNONYMS	finocchio, Florence fennel
SPREAD	Africa, Asia, Europe, North America, Oceania, South America
PLANT PARTS	fruits, seeds
TEMPERATURE	215°C / 419°F
SUBSTANCES	essential oils, fatty oil, flavonoids, acids
MEDICAL EFFECTS	carminative, mucolytic
FOLK MEDICINE	strengthening, encounters, transformation, feeling comfortable

fenugreek

LATIN	Trigonella foenum-graecum (L.)
SYNONYMS	
SPREAD	Africa, Asia, Europe, Oceania
PLANT PARTS	herb, seeds
TEMPERATURE	215°C / 419°F
SUBSTANCES	alkaloids, essential oils, bittering agent, glycosides, saponins, slime
MEDICAL EFFECTS	immuno-stimulating
FOLK MEDICINE	cleansing, encounters

field horsetail

LATIN	Equisetum arvense (L.)
SYNONYMS	common horsetail, bottlebrush, foxtail-rush, horesetail-fern, horse-pipes, meadow-pine, pine-grass, scouring-rush, snake-grass
SPREAD	Africa, Asia, Europe, North America, Oceania, South America
PLANT PARTS	herb
TEMPERATURE	230°C / 446°F
SUBSTANCES	silica, minerals, saponins
MEDICAL EFFECTS	astringent, diuretic, constricting
FOLK MEDICINE	strengthening, concentration

fly agaric

LATIN	Amanita muscaria (L.)
SYNONYMS	fly amanita
SPREAD	Africa, Asia, Europe, North America, Oceania, South America
PLANT PARTS	herb
TEMPERATURE	210°C / 410°F
SUBSTANCES	alkaloids, acids
MEDICAL EFFECTS	psychoactive
FOLK MEDICINE	trance, dream, vision , eroticizing effect

frankincense

LATIN	Boswellia sacra (Flueck.), Boswellia carteri (Birdw.), Boswellia papyrifera (Hochst.)
SYNONYMS	olibanum, elephant tree
SPREAD	Africa
PLANT PARTS	resin
TEMPERATURE	230°C / 446°F (over 300°C / 572°F)
SUBSTANCES	essential oils, bittering agent, slime
MEDICAL EFFECTS	antibacterial, anti-inflammatory, immuno-stimulating
FOLK MEDICINE	strengthening, eroticizing effect, encounters, meditation, trance, dream, vision , transformation
NOTES	Frankincense is sold in different qualities (1-4), colours (light yellow to brown), blends and provinces (Somalia, Oman, Yebahar, Ogaden, Borena etc.).

French tarragon

LATIN	Artemisia dracunculus (L.)
SYNONYMS	estragon, wild tarragon
SPREAD	Asia, Europe, North America
PLANT PARTS	herb
TEMPERATURE	230°C / 446°F
SUBSTANCES	essential oils, flavonoids, tanning agent, coumarins, acids
MEDICAL EFFECTS	appetitstimulating
FOLK MEDICINE	eroticizing effect, transformation

Fuller's teasel

LATIN	Dipsacus sylvestris (Huds.)
SYNONYMS	wild teasel
SPREAD	Europe
PLANT PARTS	herb, root
TEMPERATURE	230°C / 446°F
SUBSTANCES	bittering agent, tanning agent, saponins
MEDICAL EFFECTS	antibacterial, immuno-stimulating, pain-relieving
FOLK MEDICINE	protection, eroticizing effect, transformation, concentration, encounters, feeling comfortable

fumitory

LATIN	Fumaria officinalis (L.)
SYNONYMS	drug fumitory, earth smoke
SPREAD	Africa, Asia, Europe, North America, Oceania, South America
PLANT PARTS	herb
TEMPERATURE	225°C / 437°F
SUBSTANCES	alkaloids, bittering agent, flavonoids, slime
MEDICAL EFFECTS	aphrodisiac effect, diuretic, antispasmodic
FOLK MEDICINE	cleansing, strengthening, eroticizing effect, encounters, meditation, transformation

galanga

LATIN	Kaempferia galanga (L.)
SYNONYMS	kencur, aromatic ginger, sand ginger, cutcherry, resurrection lily
SPREAD	Asia, Europe
PLANT PARTS	root
TEMPERATURE	200°C / 392°F
SUBSTANCES	essential oils, flavonoids
MEDICAL EFFECTS	antibacterial, antioxidant , antiviral, anti-carcinogenic
FOLK MEDICINE	cleansing, concentration, encounters, feeling comfortable, eroticizing effect

galbanum

LATIN	Ferula galbaniflua (Boiss. & Buhse), Ferula gummosa (Boiss.)
SYNONYMS	giants fennel
SPREAD	Asia, Europe
PLANT PARTS	coal particles
TEMPERATURE	180°C / 356°F (max. 260°C / 500°F)
SUBSTANCES	essential oils
MEDICAL EFFECTS	anti-inflammatory
FOLK MEDICINE	meditation, transformation

garden angelica

LATIN	Angelica archangelica (L.)
SYNONYMS	angelica, Holy Ghost, wild celery, Norwegian angelica
SPREAD	Asia, Europe, North America
PLANT PARTS	blossoms, fruits, seeds, root
TEMPERATURE	200°C / 392°F
SUBSTANCES	essential oils, bittering agent, coumarins, acids
MEDICAL EFFECTS	appetitstimulating, antispasmodic, digestive
FOLK MEDICINE	feeling comfortable, concentration, meditation, encounters, transformation, eroticizing effect

garden asparagus

LATIN	Asparagus officinalis (L.)
SYNONYMS	wild asparagus
SPREAD	Asia, Europe, North America, South America
PLANT PARTS	herb, seeds, root
TEMPERATURE	220°C / 428°F
SUBSTANCES	bittering agent, fatty oil, flavonoids, tanning agent, minerals, acids
MEDICAL EFFECTS	appetitstimulating, diuretic
FOLK MEDICINE	transformation, feeling comfortable, concentration, meditation, eroticizing effect, encounters

garden chervil

LATIN	Anthriscus cerefolium (Hoffm.)
SYNONYMS	French parsley
SPREAD	Europe
PLANT PARTS	leaves, fruits, seeds
TEMPERATURE	210°C / 410°F
SUBSTANCES	essential oils, bittering agent, flavonoids
MEDICAL EFFECTS	diuretic, digestive, constricting
FOLK MEDICINE	protection, strengthening, feeling comfortable, trance, dream, vision , concentration

garden lovage

LATIN	Levisticum officinale (W.D.J. Koch)
SYNONYMS	
SPREAD	Asia, Europe
PLANT PARTS	leaves, seeds, root
TEMPERATURE	215°C / 419°F
SUBSTANCES	essential oils, coumarins
MEDICAL EFFECTS	antiseptic
FOLK MEDICINE	protection, strengthening, transformation, feeling comfortable, encounters, eroticizing effect, meditation

garden nasturtium

LATIN	Tropaeolum majus (L.)
SYNONYMS	Indian cress, monks cress
SPREAD	Asia, Europe, North America, Oceania, South America
PLANT PARTS	herb
TEMPERATURE	190°C / 374°F
SUBSTANCES	glycosides, acids
MEDICAL EFFECTS	antibacterial, antimycotic, antiviral
FOLK MEDICINE	protection, eroticizing effect, concentration, transformation

garden thyme

LATIN	Thymus vulgaris (L.)
SYNONYMS	common thyme, German thyme
SPREAD	Europe
PLANT PARTS	herb
TEMPERATURE	240°C / 464°F
SUBSTANCES	essential oils, bittering agent, flavonoids, tanning agent, saponins
MEDICAL EFFECTS	antibacterial, calming, anti-inflammatory, antipyretic, antispasmodic, digestive
FOLK MEDICINE	cleansing, strengthening, transformation, meditation, concentration, eroticizing effect

garlic

LATIN	Allium sativum (L.)
SYNONYMS	cultivated garlic, curl's treacke, clown's treacle, poorman's treacle
SPREAD	Africa, Asia, Europe, North America, Oceania, South America
PLANT PARTS	root
TEMPERATURE	215°C / 419°F
SUBSTANCES	essential oils, saponins
MEDICAL EFFECTS	anti-thrombotic, digestive
FOLK MEDICINE	protection, encounters, concentration, meditation

garlic mustard

LATIN	Arabis petiolata (M. Bieb.), Alliaria petiolata (Cavara & Grande)
SYNONYMS	Jack-by-the-hedge, garlic root, hedge garlic, sauce-alone, Jack-in-the-bush, penny hedge, poor man's mustard
SPREAD	Africa, Asia, Europe, North America, South America
PLANT PARTS	herb
TEMPERATURE	200°C / 392°F
SUBSTANCES	essential oils, flavonoids, glycosides
MEDICAL EFFECTS	digestive
FOLK MEDICINE	transformation

ginger

LATIN	Zingiber officinale (Roscoe)
SYNONYMS	
SPREAD	Africa, Asia, Europe, North America, Oceania, South America
PLANT PARTS	root
TEMPERATURE	250°C / 482°F
SUBSTANCES	essential oils, acids
MEDICAL EFFECTS	antispasmodic
FOLK MEDICINE	eroticizing effect, encounters, concentration

ginkgo

LATIN	Ginkgo biloba (L.)
SYNONYMS	maidenhair tree
SPREAD	Africa, Asia, Europe, North America, Oceania, South America
PLANT PARTS	leaves
TEMPERATURE	190°C / 374°F
SUBSTANCES	essential oils, fatty oil, flavonoids, acids
MEDICAL EFFECTS	memory-strengthening
FOLK MEDICINE	eroticizing effect

glossy eyebright

LATIN	Euphrasia officinalis (L.)
SYNONYMS	eyewort
SPREAD	Europe
PLANT PARTS	herb
TEMPERATURE	215°C / 419°F
SUBSTANCES	essential oils, tanning agent, glycosides
MEDICAL EFFECTS	anti-inflammatory
FOLK MEDICINE	meditation, eroticizing effect

golden feverfew

LATIN	Tanacetum parthenium (Sch. Bip.), Chrysanthemum parthenium (Bernh.)
SYNONYMS	bachelor's buttons, featherfew,
SPREAD	Asia, Europe, North America, Oceania, South America
PLANT PARTS	herb
TEMPERATURE	215°C / 419°F
SUBSTANCES	essential oils, tanning agent, acids
MEDICAL EFFECTS	antispasmodic, anti-carcinogenic
FOLK MEDICINE	meditation, encounters, transformation, eroticizing effect

goos grass

LATIN	Galium aparine (L.)
SYNONYMS	cleavers herb, clivers, catch-weed bedstraw, stickyweed, robin-run-the-hedge, sticky willy, sticky willow, stickyjack, stickeljack, grip grass,
SPREAD	Africa, Asia, Europe, North America, Oceania, South America
PLANT PARTS	herb
TEMPERATURE	210°C / 410°F
SUBSTANCES	glycosides, saponins, acids
MEDICAL EFFECTS	anti-inflammatory
FOLK MEDICINE	eroticizing effect, transformation

gorse

LATIN	Ulex europaeus (L.)
SYNONYMS	common gorse, furze, whin
SPREAD	Africa, Asia, Europe, North America, Oceania, South America
PLANT PARTS	blossoms
TEMPERATURE	235°C / 455°F
SUBSTANCES	flavonoids
MEDICAL EFFECTS	wound-healing
FOLK MEDICINE	meditation

grapefruit

LATIN	Citrus paradisi (Macfad.)
SYNONYMS	
SPREAD	Africa, Asia, Europe, North America, Oceania, South America
PLANT PARTS	fruit peel
TEMPERATURE	215°C / 419°F
SUBSTANCES	essential oils, flavonoids, coumarins, acids
MEDICAL EFFECTS	intentsifying
FOLK MEDICINE	cleansing, encounters, concentration

grapple plant

LATIN	Harpagophytum procumbens
SYNONYMS	devil's claw, wood spider
SPREAD	Africa
PLANT PARTS	root
TEMPERATURE	210°C / 410°F
SUBSTANCES	essential oils, flavonoids, glycosides, acids
MEDICAL EFFECTS	appetitstimulating, anti-inflammatory
FOLK MEDICINE	cleansing, meditation, encounters, eroticizing effect, concentration

graveyard moss

LATIN	Euphorbia cyparissias (L.)
SYNONYMS	graveyard-weed, quack salvers-grass, salvers spurge, cypress spurge
SPREAD	Asia, Europe
PLANT PARTS	herb
TEMPERATURE	215°C / 419°F
SUBSTANCES	essential oils, flavonoids
MEDICAL EFFECTS	antibacterial
FOLK MEDICINE	protection, transformation
NOTES	The juice is toxic and damage the skin.

gray santolina

LATIN	Santolina chamaecyparissus (L.)
SYNONYMS	lavender-cotton, cotton lavender
SPREAD	Europe
PLANT PARTS	herb
TEMPERATURE	220°C / 428°F
SUBSTANCES	essential oils, bittering agent, tanning agent
MEDICAL EFFECTS	antibacterial, disinfectant, relaxing
FOLK MEDICINE	protection, strengthening, transformation, meditation, concentration, eroticizing effect
NOTES	Also suitable as insect repellent.

great burdock

LATIN	Arctium lappa (L.)
SYNONYMS	edible burdock, cockle-button, cuckold, gobo, harlock, lappa, beggar's buttons, thorny burr, happy major
SPREAD	Africa, Asia, Europe, North America, Oceania, South America
PLANT PARTS	seeds, root
TEMPERATURE	225°C / 437°F
SUBSTANCES	essential oils, fatty oil, acids
MEDICAL EFFECTS	antibacterial
FOLK MEDICINE	feeling comfortable, concentration, eroticizing effect, encounters

greater plantain

LATIN	Plantago major (L.)
SYNONYMS	white man's foot, broadleaf plantain, cart-track-plant
SPREAD	Africa, Asia, Europe, North America, Oceania, South America
PLANT PARTS	herb, seeds
TEMPERATURE	210°C / 410°F
SUBSTANCES	tanning agent, slime
MEDICAL EFFECTS	antibacterial, astringent, mucolytic
FOLK MEDICINE	cleansing, eroticizing effect, encounters, meditation, transformation

ground ivy

LATIN	Glechoma hederacea (L.)
SYNONYMS	gill-over-the-ground, creeping charlie, alehoof, tunhoof, catsfoot, field-balm, runaway-robin, creeping jenny
SPREAD	Africa, Asia, Europe, North America, Oceania, South America
PLANT PARTS	herb
TEMPERATURE	220°C / 428°F
SUBSTANCES	essential oils, bittering agent, flavonoids, tanning agent, saponins, acids
MEDICAL EFFECTS	antibacterial, anti-inflammatory, anti-carcinogenic
FOLK MEDICINE	protection, strengthening, transformation, meditation, encounters, concentration, eroticizing effect

guaiacum

LATIN	Guaiacum officinale, G. sanctum, Bulnesia sarmienti (L.)
SYNONYMS	lignum-vitae, guaiacwood
SPREAD	South America
PLANT PARTS	resin, wood
TEMPERATURE	250°C / 482°F (over 300°C / 572°F)
SUBSTANCES	essential oils, acids
MEDICAL EFFECTS	cough suppressant
FOLK MEDICINE	feeling comfortable

guarana

LATIN	Paullinia cupana (Kunth)
SYNONYMS	
SPREAD	South America
PLANT PARTS	seeds
TEMPERATURE	215°C / 419°F
SUBSTANCES	alkaloids, tanning agent, minerals, saponins
MEDICAL EFFECTS	dehydrating, antipyretic
FOLK MEDICINE	encounters, feeling comfortable

guelder-rose

LATIN	Viburnum opulus (L.)
SYNONYMS	crampbark
SPREAD	Asia, Europe, North America
PLANT PARTS	bark
TEMPERATURE	205°C / 401°F
SUBSTANCES	tanning agent, glycosides, coumarins, acids
MEDICAL EFFECTS	antispasmodic
FOLK MEDICINE	eroticizing effect, meditation

guggul

LATIN	Commiphora wightii (Bhandari), Balsamodendrum wightii (Arn.)
SYNONYMS	Indian bdellium-tree, gugal
SPREAD	Asia
PLANT PARTS	resin
TEMPERATURE	260°C / 500°F (over 300°C / 572°F)
SUBSTANCES	essential oils
MEDICAL EFFECTS	decongestant, appetite-suppressing
FOLK MEDICINE	eroticizing effect, meditation

gum arabic tree

LATIN	Acacia senegal (Willd.), Mimosa senegal (L.)
SYNONYMS	gum acacia, Senegal gum, Sudan gum arabic, kher, khor
SPREAD	Africa
PLANT PARTS	resin
TEMPERATURE	255°C / 491°F (over 300°C / 572°F)
SUBSTANCES	tanning agent, acids
MEDICAL EFFECTS	dehydrating
FOLK MEDICINE	feeling comfortable

gum rockrose

LATIN	Cistus ladanifer (L.)
SYNONYMS	laudanum, labdanum, common gum cistus, brown-eyed rockrose
SPREAD	Africa, Asia
PLANT PARTS	leaves, blossoms, resin
TEMPERATURE	220°C / 428°F
SUBSTANCES	essential oils, flavonoids, tanning agent
MEDICAL EFFECTS	antiviral, anti-inflammatory, immuno-stimulating, wound-healing
FOLK MEDICINE	meditation, eroticizing effect, encounters, concentration, transformation, feeling comfortable

gypsywort

LATIN	Lycopus europaeus (L.)
SYNONYMS	European bugleweed, European water horehound
SPREAD	Asia, Europe, North America
PLANT PARTS	herb
TEMPERATURE	220°C / 428°F
SUBSTANCES	essential oils, flavonoids, tanning agent, acids
MEDICAL EFFECTS	calming, pain-relieving
FOLK MEDICINE	concentration, transformation, eroticizing effect

hawthorn

LATIN	Crataegus (L.)
SYNONYMS	thornapple may-tree, whitethorn, hawberry, red haw
SPREAD	Asia, Europe, North America
PLANT PARTS	blossoms, fruits, wood
TEMPERATURE	200°C / 392°F
SUBSTANCES	flavonoids, tanning agent
MEDICAL EFFECTS	digestive
FOLK MEDICINE	strengthening, eroticizing effect, encounters, feeling comfortable, transformation

hazel

LATIN	Corylus avellana (L.)
SYNONYMS	common hazel, American hazelnut, European filbert
SPREAD	Asia, Europe, North America
PLANT PARTS	leaves
TEMPERATURE	225°C / 437°F
SUBSTANCES	tanning agent, acids
MEDICAL EFFECTS	anti-inflammatory, labor-inducing
FOLK MEDICINE	encounters, transformation, eroticizing effect

hemp

LATIN	Cannabis sativa (L.), Cannabis indica (Lam.), Cannabis ruderalis (Janisch.)
SYNONYMS	marijuana, hashish, kief, gallow-grass, grass, neck-weed, red-root, pot
SPREAD	Africa, Asia, Europe, North America, Oceania, South America
PLANT PARTS	blossoms
TEMPERATURE	220°C / 428°F
SUBSTANCES	essential oils, flavonoids
MEDICAL EFFECTS	aphrodisiac effect, calming, blood pressure-reducing, antispasmodic, psychoactive
FOLK MEDICINE	encounters, trance, dream, vision

henbane

LATIN	Hyoscyamus niger (L.)
SYNONYMS	black henbane, stinking nightshade
SPREAD	Africa, Asia, Europe
PLANT PARTS	herb
TEMPERATURE	230°C / 446°F
SUBSTANCES	alkaloids
MEDICAL EFFECTS	antispasmodic, psychoactive, pain-relieving
FOLK MEDICINE	trance, dream, vision , encounters, eroticizing effect

henna

LATIN	Lawsonia inermis (L.)
SYNONYMS	hina, mignonette tree, Egyptian privet
SPREAD	Africa, Asia
PLANT PARTS	leaves
TEMPERATURE	225°C / 437°F
SUBSTANCES	tanning agent, acids
MEDICAL EFFECTS	antibacterial
FOLK MEDICINE	protection, transformation, concentration

herb-Robert

LATIN	Geranium robertianum (L.)
SYNONYMS	Robert geranium, red Robin, death come quickly, storksbill, dove's foot, crow's foot
SPREAD	Africa, Asia, Europe, North America
PLANT PARTS	herb
TEMPERATURE	225°C / 437°F
SUBSTANCES	essential oils, bittering agent, tanning agent
MEDICAL EFFECTS	dehydrating
FOLK MEDICINE	feeling comfortable, eroticizing effect

high mallow

LATIN	Malva sylvestris (L.)
SYNONYMS	cheeses, tall mallow
SPREAD	Africa, Asia, Europe
PLANT PARTS	leaves, blossoms, seeds, root
TEMPERATURE	215°C / 419°F
SUBSTANCES	essential oils, flavonoids, tanning agent, slime
MEDICAL EFFECTS	anti-inflammatory, cough suppressant, pain-relieving
FOLK MEDICINE	protection, encounters, eroticizing effect, feeling comfortable, meditation, transformation

Himalayan balsam

LATIN	Impatiens glandulifera (Royle)
SYNONYMS	ornamental jewelweed, Indian balsam, kiss-me-on-the-mountain, policeman's helmet, Bobby tops, copper tops, gnome's hatstand
SPREAD	Asia, Europe, North America
PLANT PARTS	herb
TEMPERATURE	200°C / 392°F
SUBSTANCES	bittering agent, tanning agent, glycosides
MEDICAL EFFECTS	antibacterial, diuretic
FOLK MEDICINE	transformation, meditation, eroticizing effect

Himalayan rhododendron

LATIN	Rhododendron anthopogon (D. Don)
SYNONYMS	
SPREAD	Asia
PLANT PARTS	herb, root
TEMPERATURE	230°C / 446°F (max. 260°C / 500°F)
SUBSTANCES	essential oils, glycosides
MEDICAL EFFECTS	diuretic
FOLK MEDICINE	strengthening, transformation, encounters, meditation, eroticizing effect

hollowstem burnet saxifrage

LATIN	Pimpinella major (Huds.)
SYNONYMS	greater burnet-saxifrage
SPREAD	Asia, Europe, North America
PLANT PARTS	root
TEMPERATURE	215°C / 419°F
SUBSTANCES	essential oils, tanning agent, coumarins, saponins
MEDICAL EFFECTS	antibacterial, astringent, anti-inflammatory, diuretic, mucolytic
FOLK MEDICINE	concentration, encounters, meditation, feeling comfortable, eroticizing effect

holy basil

LATIN	Ocimum tenuiflorum (L.)
SYNONYMS	tulsi, tulasi
SPREAD	Asia, Oceania
PLANT PARTS	herb
TEMPERATURE	240°C / 464°F
SUBSTANCES	essential oils, flavonoids
MEDICAL EFFECTS	antibacterial
FOLK MEDICINE	protection, transformation
NOTES	Tulsi is a sacred plant in India.

holy wood

LATIN	Bursera graveolens (Triana & Planch.B.), Elaphrium graveolens (Kunth), Terebinthus graveolens (Rose)
SYNONYMS	palo santo
SPREAD	North America, South America
PLANT PARTS	resin, wood
TEMPERATURE	220°C / 428°F
SUBSTANCES	essential oils, bittering agent, acids
MEDICAL EFFECTS	relaxing
FOLK MEDICINE	protection, strengthening, meditation, feeling comfortable, eroticizing effect

horehound

LATIN	Marrubium vulgare (L.)
SYNONYMS	white horehound, hound-bane, marrube, marvel
SPREAD	Europe, North America, Oceania, South America
PLANT PARTS	herb
TEMPERATURE	230°C / 446°F
SUBSTANCES	essential oils, bittering agent, flavonoids, tanning agent, acids
MEDICAL EFFECTS	appetitstimulating, digestive
FOLK MEDICINE	eroticizing effect, transformation, encounters

horse-chestnut

LATIN	Aesculus hippocastanum (L.)
SYNONYMS	European horse-chestnut, conker tree
SPREAD	Asia, Europe, North America, Oceania
PLANT PARTS	leaves, blossoms, fruits, seeds, bark
TEMPERATURE	200°C / 392°F
SUBSTANCES	bittering agent, tanning agent, glycosides, coumarins, saponins, acids
MEDICAL EFFECTS	astringent, anti-inflammatory
FOLK MEDICINE	concentration, transformation, meditation, eroticizing effect, encounters, feeling comfortable

horseradish

LATIN	Armoracia rusticana (G. Gaertn., B. Mey. & Scherb.)
SYNONYMS	Red-cole
SPREAD	Africa, Asia, Europe
PLANT PARTS	root
TEMPERATURE	190°C / 374°F
SUBSTANCES	essential oils, flavonoids, glycosides, minerals
MEDICAL EFFECTS	antibacterial, antipyretic, antispasmodic, pain-relieving, digestive
FOLK MEDICINE	concentration, encounters, eroticizing effect, meditation

houndstongue

LATIN	Cynoglossum officinale (L.)
SYNONYMS	gypsyflower, houndstooth, dog's tongue, rats and mice
SPREAD	Asia, Europe, North America
PLANT PARTS	herb, root
TEMPERATURE	225°C / 437°F
SUBSTANCES	alkaloids, essential oils, tanning agent, slime
MEDICAL EFFECTS	cough suppressant, wound-healing
FOLK MEDICINE	encounters, eroticizing effect, feeling comfortable, meditation, transformation

huisache

LATIN	Acacia farnesiana (Willd.), Vachellia farnesiana (Wight & Arn.), Mimosa farnesiana (L.)
SYNONYMS	mimosa farnesiana, needle bush, acacia farnesiana, sweet acacia, aromo
SPREAD	Africa, Asia, Europe, North America, Oceania, South America
PLANT PARTS	resin, wood
TEMPERATURE	190°C / 374°F
SUBSTANCES	tanning agent
MEDICAL EFFECTS	dehydrating
FOLK MEDICINE	feeling comfortable

hyssop

LATIN	Hyssopus officinalis (L.)
SYNONYMS	
SPREAD	Africa, Asia, Europe
PLANT PARTS	leaves
TEMPERATURE	210°C / 410°F
SUBSTANCES	essential oils, tanning agent, glycosides, acids
MEDICAL EFFECTS	anti-inflammatory, antispasmodic, mucolytic
FOLK MEDICINE	cleansing, strengthening, eroticizing effect, meditation, concentration, transformation

Iceland moss

LATIN	Cetraria islandica (L.)
SYNONYMS	Iceland lichen
SPREAD	Europe, North America
PLANT PARTS	herb
TEMPERATURE	235°C / 455°F
SUBSTANCES	essential oils, bittering agent, acids, slime
MEDICAL EFFECTS	anti-inflammatory
FOLK MEDICINE	cleansing, meditation, concentration, eroticizing effect

Indian chrysanthemum

LATIN	Chrysanthemum indicum (L.)
SYNONYMS	Paris daisy, marguerite, marguerite daisy
SPREAD	Asia, Europe
PLANT PARTS	blossoms
TEMPERATURE	205°C / 401°F
SUBSTANCES	essential oils, glycosides
MEDICAL EFFECTS	anti-inflammatory
FOLK MEDICINE	encounters
NOTES	Use in traditional Chinese medicine.

Indian frankincense

LATIN	Boswellia serrata (Roxb. ex Colebr.)
SYNONYMS	salai, shallaki, olibanum indicum
SPREAD	Africa, Asia
PLANT PARTS	resin
TEMPERATURE	250°C / 482°F (over 300°C / 572°F)
SUBSTANCES	essential oils, acids, slime
MEDICAL EFFECTS	anti-inflammatory
FOLK MEDICINE	meditation, feeling comfortable, transformation

Indian sarsaparilla

LATIN	Hemidesmus Indicus (R. Br. ex Schult.)
SYNONYMS	
SPREAD	Asia
PLANT PARTS	root
TEMPERATURE	240°C / 464°F
SUBSTANCES	alkaloids, essential oils, flavonoids, tanning agent, coumarins, acids
MEDICAL EFFECTS	blood cleansing
FOLK MEDICINE	protection, encounters

Irish moss

LATIN	Chondrus crispus (Stackh.)
SYNONYMS	carrageen moss, Irish carraigin, little rock
SPREAD	Asia, Europe, North America
PLANT PARTS	herb
TEMPERATURE	220°C / 428°F
SUBSTANCES	bittering agent, slime
MEDICAL EFFECTS	antimicrobiologic , soothing
FOLK MEDICINE	strengthening, eroticizing effect
NOTES	May cause allergic reactions.

Java plum

LATIN	Syzygium cumini (Skeels), Myrtus cumini (L.)
SYNONYMS	jamblang, jamun, black plum, jambul, jambolan
SPREAD	Africa, Asia, North America, Oceania
PLANT PARTS	leaves, bark
TEMPERATURE	230°C / 446°F
SUBSTANCES	essential oils, tanning agent
MEDICAL EFFECTS	constricting
FOLK MEDICINE	feeling comfortable, concentration

Java tea

LATIN	Orthosiphon stamineus (Benth.)
SYNONYMS	kidney tea plant
SPREAD	Africa, Asia, Oceania
PLANT PARTS	leaves
TEMPERATURE	220°C / 428°F
SUBSTANCES	essential oils, flavonoids
MEDICAL EFFECTS	diuretic, antispasmodic
FOLK MEDICINE	concentration

kauri

LATIN	Agathis australis (Steud.)
SYNONYMS	New Zealand kauri
SPREAD	Oceania
PLANT PARTS	leaves
TEMPERATURE	220°C / 428°F
SUBSTANCES	essential oils
MEDICAL EFFECTS	antiseptic
FOLK MEDICINE	strengthening, transformation
NOTES	Kauri is very difficult to obtain.

kava

LATIN	Piper methysticum (G. Forst.)
SYNONYMS	awa, kava-kava
SPREAD	Oceania
PLANT PARTS	root
TEMPERATURE	230°C / 446°F
SUBSTANCES	alkaloids, essential oils, flavonoids, acids
MEDICAL EFFECTS	antidepressant, pain-relieving
FOLK MEDICINE	meditation, trance, dream, vision , encounters

lady's bedstraw

LATIN	Galium verum (L.)
SYNONYMS	yellow bedstraw, cheese-rennet, bed-flower, curd-wort
SPREAD	Africa, Asia, Europe, North America, Oceania
PLANT PARTS	herb
TEMPERATURE	235°C / 455°F
SUBSTANCES	flavonoids, tanning agent, glycosides, silica
MEDICAL EFFECTS	anti-inflammatory, antispasmodic, wound-healing
FOLK MEDICINE	transformation, feeling comfortable, meditation, eroticizing effect

lady's mantle

LATIN	Alchemilla mollis (L.), Alchemilla vulgaris (LT)
SYNONYMS	
SPREAD	Africa, Asia, Europe, North America, Oceania, South America
PLANT PARTS	plant
TEMPERATURE	200°C / 392°F
SUBSTANCES	essential oils, bittering agent, tanning agent, glycosides, saponins
MEDICAL EFFECTS	decongestant, calming
FOLK MEDICINE	protection, cleansing, strengthening, eroticizing effect
NOTES	It is often confused with the "ordinary piglet herb", which does not have a hollow stem.

lemon balm

LATIN	Melissa officinalis (L.)
SYNONYMS	common balm, balm mint, sweet balm, bee balm
SPREAD	Asia, Europe
PLANT PARTS	leaves
TEMPERATURE	215°C / 419°F
SUBSTANCES	essential oils, bittering agent, flavonoids, tanning agent, glycosides, saponins, slime
MEDICAL EFFECTS	antibacterial, antiviral, calming, antispasmodic, labor-inducing
FOLK MEDICINE	protection, cleansing, eroticizing effect, feeling comfortable, concentration, meditation

lemon grass

LATIN	Cymbopogon citratus (Stapf), Andropogon citratus (DC.)
SYNONYMS	oil grass, fever grass,
SPREAD	Africa, Asia, Europe, North America, Oceania, South America
PLANT PARTS	leaves
TEMPERATURE	240°C / 464°F
SUBSTANCES	essential oils, flavonoids, glycosides, saponins
MEDICAL EFFECTS	calming
FOLK MEDICINE	strengthening, feeling comfortable, concentration, eroticizing effect

linden

LATIN	Tilia (L.)
SYNONYMS	basswood, lime tree, lime bush
SPREAD	Asia, Europe, North America
PLANT PARTS	blossoms
TEMPERATURE	235°C / 455°F
SUBSTANCES	essential oils, flavonoids, tanning agent, glycosides, saponins, acids, slime
MEDICAL EFFECTS	calming, antispasmodic, mucolytic, pain-relieving
FOLK MEDICINE	cleansing, encounters, meditation, eroticizing effect

liverleaf

LATIN	Hepatica nobilis (Schreb.)
SYNONYMS	round-lobe hepatica, kidneywort, pennywort, American liverleaf
SPREAD	Asia, Europe, North America
PLANT PARTS	herb
TEMPERATURE	225°C / 437°F
SUBSTANCES	flavonoids, tanning agent, glycosides, saponins
MEDICAL EFFECTS	diuretic, wound-healing
FOLK MEDICINE	cleansing, strengthening, transformation, feeling comfortable, meditation, concentration

llima

LATIN	Sida cordifolia (L.)
SYNONYMS	ilima, bala, country mallow, heart-leaf sida, flannel weed
SPREAD	Africa, Asia, Oceania, South America
PLANT PARTS	root
TEMPERATURE	250°C / 482°F
SUBSTANCES	amphetamines, essential oils
MEDICAL EFFECTS	anti-inflammatory, antipyretic, psychoactive
FOLK MEDICINE	encounters, trance, dream, vision

locust

LATIN	Hymenaea courbaril (L.)
SYNONYMS	West Indian locust, Brazilian copal, amami-gum, stinking toe, courbaril
SPREAD	Africa, South America
PLANT PARTS	resin
TEMPERATURE	290°C / 554°F (over 300°C / 572°F)
SUBSTANCES	essential oils
MEDICAL EFFECTS	antiseptic
FOLK MEDICINE	protection, strengthening, trance, dream, vision , feeling comfortable
NOTES	This substance is extracted from the earth like amber, but is less old.

maca

LATIN	Lepidium meyenii (Walp.)
SYNONYMS	
SPREAD	South America
PLANT PARTS	root
TEMPERATURE	190°C / 374°F
SUBSTANCES	alkaloids, tanning agent, saponins, acids
MEDICAL EFFECTS	virility-enhancing
FOLK MEDICINE	encounters

mangosteen

LATIN	Garcinia mangostana (L.)
SYNONYMS	purple mangosteen
SPREAD	Africa, Asia, Oceania, South America
PLANT PARTS	peel
TEMPERATURE	215°C / 419°F
SUBSTANCES	acids
MEDICAL EFFECTS	antiallergic, antibacterial, antimycotic, antiviral, anti-inflammatory, pain-relieving, anti-carcinogenic
FOLK MEDICINE	protection, cleansing, strengthening, eroticizing effect, feeling comfortable

manna ash

LATIN	Fraxinus ornus (L.)
SYNONYMS	South European flowering ash
SPREAD	Europe
PLANT PARTS	resin
TEMPERATURE	260°C / 500°F (over 300°C / 572°F)
SUBSTANCES	essential oils
MEDICAL EFFECTS	laxative
FOLK MEDICINE	meditation

marigold

LATIN	Calendula officinalis (L.)
SYNONYMS	ruddles, English marigold, Scottish marigold, garden mariegold, pot-marigold
SPREAD	Europe
PLANT PARTS	blossoms
TEMPERATURE	210°C / 410°F
SUBSTANCES	essential oils, bittering agent, fatty oil, flavonoids, tanning agent
MEDICAL EFFECTS	anti-inflammatory, wound-healing
FOLK MEDICINE	encounters, meditation

maritime pine

LATIN	Pinus pinaster (Aiton)
SYNONYMS	cluster pine
SPREAD	Europe
PLANT PARTS	resin, needles
TEMPERATURE	210°C / 410°F (max. 260°C / 500°F)
SUBSTANCES	essential oils, acids
MEDICAL EFFECTS	anti-inflammatory
FOLK MEDICINE	protection, strengthening, meditation, eroticizing effect, feeling comfortable

marshmallow

LATIN	Althaea officinalis (L.)
SYNONYMS	marsh-mallow, common marshmallow, shrubwoods, river banks, saline soil
SPREAD	Asia, Europe
PLANT PARTS	leaves, blossoms, root
TEMPERATURE	250°C / 482°F
SUBSTANCES	essential oils, tanning agent, coumarins, saponins, acids, slime
MEDICAL EFFECTS	anti-inflammatory
FOLK MEDICINE	protection, eroticizing effect, transformation, feeling comfortable

masterwort

LATIN	Peucedanum ostruthium (W.D.J. Koch), Imperatoria ostruthium (L.)
SYNONYMS	
SPREAD	Europe, North America
PLANT PARTS	root
TEMPERATURE	220°C / 428°F
SUBSTANCES	essential oils, bittering agent, tanning agent, coumarins
MEDICAL EFFECTS	antibacterial
FOLK MEDICINE	protection, strengthening, concentration, feeling comfortable, encounters
NOTES	In the Middle Ages it was considered a panacea.

mastic tree

LATIN	Pistacia lentiscus (L.)
SYNONYMS	mastix, lentisk
SPREAD	Africa, Asia, Oceania, South America
PLANT PARTS	resin
TEMPERATURE	280°C / 536°F (over 300°C / 572°F)
SUBSTANCES	essential oils, acids
MEDICAL EFFECTS	antibacterial, antimicrobiologic , antimycotic, antiviral
FOLK MEDICINE	cleansing, strengthening, concentration, trance, dream, vision , transformation, encounters, eroticizing effect, meditation

meadowsweet

LATIN	Filipendula ulmaria (Maxim.)
SYNONYMS	mead wort, meadow queen, pride of the meadow, eadow-wort, lady of the meadow, dollof, meadsweet, bridewort
SPREAD	Asia, Europe, North America
PLANT PARTS	herb
TEMPERATURE	200°C / 392°F
SUBSTANCES	essential oils, flavonoids, tanning agent, acids
MEDICAL EFFECTS	diuretic, pain-relieving
FOLK MEDICINE	encounters, transformation

Mediterranean cypress

LATIN	Cupressus sempervirens (L.)
SYNONYMS	Italian cypress, Tuscan cypress, graveyard cypress, pencil pine
SPREAD	Africa, Europe
PLANT PARTS	leaves, fruits, seeds, needles
TEMPERATURE	220°C / 428°F
SUBSTANCES	essential oils
MEDICAL EFFECTS	antibacterial, antimicrobiologic , improving the ability to concentrate, antispasmodic
FOLK MEDICINE	concentration, eroticizing effect, transformation

Mexican tea

LATIN	Dysphania ambrosioides (Mosyakin & Clemants), Chenopodium ambrosioides (L.)
SYNONYMS	American worm-seed, strong-scented pigweed, Indian goosefoot, Jerusalem tea, Jesuit's tea, Spanish teawormseed
SPREAD	Europe, North America, South America
PLANT PARTS	herb
TEMPERATURE	220°C / 428°F
SUBSTANCES	essential oils
MEDICAL EFFECTS	digestive
FOLK MEDICINE	transformation

milk thistle

LATIN	Silybum marianum (Gaertn.)
SYNONYMS	blessed milkthistle, Marian thistle, Mary thistle, Saint Mary's thistle, Mediterranean milk thistle, variegated thistle, Scotch thistle
SPREAD	Africa, Asia, Europe, North America, Oceania, South America
PLANT PARTS	fruits, seeds
TEMPERATURE	215°C / 419°F
SUBSTANCES	fatty oil, flavonoids, acids
MEDICAL EFFECTS	detoxifying, antispasmodic
FOLK MEDICINE	encounters, feeling comfortable, transformation

mistletoe

LATIN	Viscum album (L.)
SYNONYMS	European mistletoe, common mistletoe
SPREAD	Europe, North America
PLANT PARTS	leaves
TEMPERATURE	215°C / 419°F
SUBSTANCES	bittering agent, flavonoids, saponins, acids, slime
MEDICAL EFFECTS	blood pressure-reducing, anti-carcinogenic , digestive
FOLK MEDICINE	strengthening, concentration, trance, dream, vision

mountain arnica

LATIN	Arnica montana (L.)
SYNONYMS	leopard's bane, mountain tobacco, mountain arnica, wolf's bane
SPREAD	Europe
PLANT PARTS	blossoms, root
TEMPERATURE	230°C / 446°F
SUBSTANCES	essential oils, bittering agent, flavonoids
MEDICAL EFFECTS	decongestant, antiseptic, anti-inflammatory, immuno-stimulating
FOLK MEDICINE	cleansing, eroticizing effect, meditation, concentration, feeling comfortable

mountain ash

LATIN	Sorbus aucuparia (L.)
SYNONYMS	rowan
SPREAD	Africa, Asia, Europe
PLANT PARTS	leaves, bark
TEMPERATURE	205°C / 401°F
SUBSTANCES	anthranoids, essential oils, bittering agent, flavonoids, tanning agent, coumarins, slime
MEDICAL EFFECTS	laxative, lymph-cleansing
FOLK MEDICINE	protection, meditation, feeling comfortable, eroticizing effect, concentration, transformation

mountain pomegranate

LATIN	Catunaregam spinosa (Tirveng.), Gardenia spinosa (Thunb.)
SYNONYMS	karegida
SPREAD	Asia
PLANT PARTS	fruits, seeds, nuts
TEMPERATURE	240°C / 464°F
SUBSTANCES	alkaloids, essential oils
MEDICAL EFFECTS	calming
FOLK MEDICINE	eroticizing effect, meditation

mouse-ear-hawkweed

LATIN	Pilosella officinarum (Vaill.), Hieracium pilosella (L.)
SYNONYMS	Mouse-ear, felon-herb, mouse-bloodwort, mouse-ear hawkweed, mouse-eared hawkweed
SPREAD	Asia, Europe, North America, Oceania
PLANT PARTS	leaves
TEMPERATURE	230°C / 446°F
SUBSTANCES	bittering agent, flavonoids, tanning agent, coumarins
MEDICAL EFFECTS	dehydrating
FOLK MEDICINE	strengthening, feeling comfortable, meditation

mugwort

LATIN	Artemisia vulgaris (L.)
SYNONYMS	common wormwood, felon herb, chrysanthemum weed, wild wormwood, old Uncle Henry, sailor's tobacco, naughty man, old man, St. John's plant
SPREAD	Africa, Europe
PLANT PARTS	herb
TEMPERATURE	230°C / 446°F
SUBSTANCES	essential oils, bittering agent, tanning agent, coumarins
MEDICAL EFFECTS	appetitstimulating, nervine, labor-inducing
FOLK MEDICINE	protection, cleansing, strengthening, trance, dream, vision , transformation, eroticizing effect
NOTES	Mugwort used to be considered the remedy for midwives.

musk mallow

LATIN	Abelmoschus moschatus (Medik.), Hibiscus moschatus (L.)
SYNONYMS	abelmosk, ambrette seeds, annual hibiscus, bamia moschata, muskdana, musk okra, musk seed, ornamental okra, rose mallow seed, tropical jewel hibiscus, yorka okra
SPREAD	Asia
PLANT PARTS	fruits, seeds, grains
TEMPERATURE	220°C / 428°F
SUBSTANCES	essential oils, fatty oil, flavonoids, glycosides
MEDICAL EFFECTS	detoxifying
FOLK MEDICINE	encounters
NOTES	Used in India against snake bites.

myrrh

LATIN	Commiphora myrrha (Engl.)
SYNONYMS	African myrrh, herabol myrrh, Somali myrrhor, common myrrh, gum myrrh
SPREAD	Africa, Asia, Oceania, South America
PLANT PARTS	resin
TEMPERATURE	280°C / 536°F (over 300°C / 572°F)
SUBSTANCES	essential oils, slime
MEDICAL EFFECTS	dehydrating, warming, psychoactive, wound-healing, constricting
FOLK MEDICINE	cleansing, strengthening, feeling comfortable, encounters

myrtle

LATIN	Myrtus communis (L.)
SYNONYMS	Greek myrtle, Swedish myrtle, Indian buchu
SPREAD	Africa, Asia, Europe
PLANT PARTS	leaves
TEMPERATURE	210°C / 410°F
SUBSTANCES	essential oils
MEDICAL EFFECTS	antimycotic, anti-inflammatory
FOLK MEDICINE	strengthening, concentration, eroticizing effect
NOTES	One of the 4 holy Jewish plants (myrtle, date palm, willow, lemon).

nard

LATIN	Nardostachys jatamansi (DC.)
SYNONYMS	nardin, muskroot
SPREAD	Asia
PLANT PARTS	root
TEMPERATURE	200°C / 392°F
SUBSTANCES	essential oils
MEDICAL EFFECTS	calming
FOLK MEDICINE	eroticizing effect, meditation

neem

LATIN	Azadirachta indica (A. Juss.), Melia azadirachta (L.)
SYNONYMS	nimtree, Indian lilac
SPREAD	Africa, Asia, Oceania, South America
PLANT PARTS	leaves
TEMPERATURE	225°C / 437°F
SUBSTANCES	tanning agent
MEDICAL EFFECTS	antibacterial, antimycotic, antiviral
FOLK MEDICINE	concentration, meditation

New Jersey Tea

LATIN	Ceanothus americanus (L.)
SYNONYMS	Jersey tea ceanothus, red root, mountain sweet, wild snowball
SPREAD	North America
PLANT PARTS	root
TEMPERATURE	245°C / 473°F
SUBSTANCES	alkaloids, tanning agent
MEDICAL EFFECTS	anti-inflammatory
FOLK MEDICINE	eroticizing effect, encounters

northern Labrador tea

LATIN	Ledum palustre (L.), Rhododendron tomentosum (Harmaja), Rhododendron palustre (Turcz.)
SYNONYMS	marsh Labrador tea, wild rosemary
SPREAD	Asia, Europe, North America
PLANT PARTS	herb
TEMPERATURE	225°C / 437°F
SUBSTANCES	essential oils, flavonoids, tanning agent, glycosides
MEDICAL EFFECTS	antibacterial, diuretic, antispasmodic, psychoactive
FOLK MEDICINE	transformation, meditation, eroticizing effect

Norway spruce

LATIN	Picea Abies (H. Karst.)
SYNONYMS	
SPREAD	Africa, Asia, Europe, North America, Oceania, South America
PLANT PARTS	resin, ,needles
TEMPERATURE	260°C / 500°F (max. 290°C / 554°F)
SUBSTANCES	essential oils, tanning agent, glycosides
MEDICAL EFFECTS	antibacterial, anti-inflammatory
FOLK MEDICINE	protection, strengthening, eroticizing effect, transformation, meditation

nutmeg

LATIN	Myristica fragrans (Houtt.)
SYNONYMS	evergreen tree
SPREAD	Africa, Asia, Oceania, South America
PLANT PARTS	fruits, seeds, nuts
TEMPERATURE	225°C / 437°F
SUBSTANCES	essential oils, fatty oil
MEDICAL EFFECTS	antibacterial, anti-inflammatory, antispasmodic, psychoactive
FOLK MEDICINE	encounters, trance, dream, vision , eroticizing effect, transformation

oakmoss

LATIN	Evernia prunastri (Ach.), Lichen prunastri L.
SYNONYMS	Irish lichens
SPREAD	Europe
PLANT PARTS	herb
TEMPERATURE	225°C / 437°F
SUBSTANCES	essential oils, acids
MEDICAL EFFECTS	antibacterial
FOLK MEDICINE	transformation
NOTES	May cause allergic reactions.

official burnet

LATIN	Sanguisorba officinalis (L.)
SYNONYMS	great burnet
SPREAD	Asia, Europe, North America
PLANT PARTS	herb, root
TEMPERATURE	215°C / 419°F
SUBSTANCES	flavonoids, tanning agent, glycosides
MEDICAL EFFECTS	astringent
FOLK MEDICINE	meditation, encounters

old man's beard

LATIN	Usnea barbata (Weber ex F.H. Wigg.), Lichen barbatus (L.)
SYNONYMS	beard lichen, tree moss
SPREAD	Africa, Asia, Europe, North America, Oceania, South America
PLANT PARTS	herb
TEMPERATURE	220°C / 428°F
SUBSTANCES	acids
MEDICAL EFFECTS	antibacterial
FOLK MEDICINE	strengthening, transformation

olive

LATIN	Olea europaea (L.)
SYNONYMS	
SPREAD	Asia, Europe, North America, South America
PLANT PARTS	leaves
TEMPERATURE	210°C / 410°F
SUBSTANCES	bittering agent, acids
MEDICAL EFFECTS	anti-inflammatory
FOLK MEDICINE	cleansing, concentration, eroticizing effect

onion

LATIN	Allium cepa (L.), Cepa vulgaris (Garsault), Kepa esculenta (Raf.), Porrum cepa (Rchb.)
SYNONYMS	bulb onion, common onion
SPREAD	Africa, Asia, Europe, North America, Oceania, South America
PLANT PARTS	root
TEMPERATURE	180°C / 356°F
SUBSTANCES	essential oils, tanning agent, glycosides, silica, minerals, acids
MEDICAL EFFECTS	antibacterial, diuretic
FOLK MEDICINE	concentration, encounters, feeling comfortable, eroticizing effect

opopanax

LATIN	Commiphora spp.
SYNONYMS	
SPREAD	Africa, Europe
PLANT PARTS	resin
TEMPERATURE	280°C / 536°F (over 300°C / 572°F)
SUBSTANCES	essential oils
MEDICAL EFFECTS	anti-inflammatory
FOLK MEDICINE	strengthening, feeling comfortable, meditation

orange

LATIN	Citrus sinensis (Osbeck), Citrus aurantium var. sinensis (L.)
SYNONYMS	sweet orange, blood orange, navel orange
SPREAD	Africa, Asia, Oceania, South America
PLANT PARTS	fruits, seeds, peel
TEMPERATURE	195°C / 383°F
SUBSTANCES	essential oils, flavonoids, acids
MEDICAL EFFECTS	antibacterial, anti-inflammatory, anti-carcinogenic , constricting
FOLK MEDICINE	cleansing, trance, dream, vision , eroticizing effect, transformation, encounters, concentration, feeling comfortable
NOTES	For leaves the smoking temperature is 215°.

oregano

LATIN	Origanum vulgare (L.)
SYNONYMS	wild marjoram, pot marjoram
SPREAD	Africa, Asia, Europe, North America, Oceania, South America
PLANT PARTS	leaves
TEMPERATURE	235°C / 455°F
SUBSTANCES	essential oils, bittering agent, flavonoids, tanning agent
MEDICAL EFFECTS	anti-inflammatory, digestive
FOLK MEDICINE	concentration, eroticizing effect, feeling comfortable, transformation

oval-leaf knotweed

LATIN	Polygonum arenastrum (Boreau)
SYNONYMS	equal-leaved knotgrass, common knotweed, prostrate knotweed, mat grass, stone grass, wiregrass, door weed
SPREAD	Africa, Asia, Europe, North America, Oceania, South America
PLANT PARTS	herb
TEMPERATURE	200°C / 392°F
SUBSTANCES	essential oils, flavonoids, tanning agent, silica, coumarins, minerals, slime
MEDICAL EFFECTS	astringent, anti-inflammatory, diuretic, soporific, wound-healing
FOLK MEDICINE	meditation, transformation, eroticizing effect, feeling comfortable, concentration, encounters

papaya

LATIN	Carica papaya (L.)
SYNONYMS	melon-tree, pawpaw
SPREAD	Africa, Asia, Oceania, South America
PLANT PARTS	seeds
TEMPERATURE	190°C / 374°F
SUBSTANCES	alkaloids, saponins
MEDICAL EFFECTS	digestive
FOLK MEDICINE	feeling comfortable

parsley

LATIN	Petroselinum crispum (Fuss)
SYNONYMS	garden parsley
SPREAD	Africa, Asia, Europe, North America, Oceania, South America
PLANT PARTS	herb
TEMPERATURE	215°C / 419°F
SUBSTANCES	essential oils, flavonoids, glycosides, acids
MEDICAL EFFECTS	diuretic
FOLK MEDICINE	cleansing, transformation, meditation

patchouli

LATIN	Pogostemon cablin (Benth.)
SYNONYMS	patchouly
SPREAD	Asia
PLANT PARTS	leaves
TEMPERATURE	210°C / 410°F
SUBSTANCES	essential oils
MEDICAL EFFECTS	calming
FOLK MEDICINE	cleansing, encounters, eroticizing effect

pedunculate oak

LATIN	Quercus robur (L.)
SYNONYMS	common oak, European oak, English oak, truffle oak
SPREAD	Asia, Europe
PLANT PARTS	leaves, bark
TEMPERATURE	230°C / 446°F
SUBSTANCES	bittering agent, tanning agent, acids
MEDICAL EFFECTS	antibacterial, dehydrating, astringent, anti-inflammatory
FOLK MEDICINE	cleansing, strengthening, concentration, eroticizing effect, feeling comfortable, transformation

peony

LATIN	Paeonia officinalis (L.) (L.)
SYNONYMS	garden peony, marshmallow button
SPREAD	Asia, Europe
PLANT PARTS	blossoms, seeds, root
TEMPERATURE	200°C / 392°F
SUBSTANCES	essential oils, tanning agent, glycosides, acids
MEDICAL EFFECTS	calming, antispasmodic
FOLK MEDICINE	encounters, feeling comfortable, meditation, transformation, concentration, eroticizing effect
NOTES	Use in traditional Chinese medicine.

peppermint

LATIN	Mentha x piperita (L.)
SYNONYMS	
SPREAD	Africa, Asia, Europe, North America, Oceania, South America
PLANT PARTS	leaves, herb
TEMPERATURE	240°C / 464°F
SUBSTANCES	essential oils, bittering agent, flavonoids, tanning agent
MEDICAL EFFECTS	antibacterial, antiviral, antispasmodic
FOLK MEDICINE	cleansing, strengthening, concentration, meditation, transformation, eroticizing effect

perfoliate honeysuckle

LATIN	Lonicera caprifolia (L.)
SYNONYMS	Italian honeysuckle, Italian woodbine, goat-leaf honeysuckle, perfoliate woodbine
SPREAD	Asia, Europe, South America
PLANT PARTS	blossoms
TEMPERATURE	210°C / 410°F
SUBSTANCES	alkaloids, essential oils, tanning agent, glycosides, saponins, slime
MEDICAL EFFECTS	diuretic
FOLK MEDICINE	transformation

pichi

LATIN	Fabiana imbricata (Ruiz & Pav.)
SYNONYMS	pichi-pichi
SPREAD	South America
PLANT PARTS	wood, herb
TEMPERATURE	220°C / 428°F
SUBSTANCES	alkaloids, essential oils, bittering agent, flavonoids, glycosides, coumarins
MEDICAL EFFECTS	stimulating
FOLK MEDICINE	protection, strengthening, eroticizing effect, meditation
NOTES	This substance is difficult to obtain in Europe.

plumbago

LATIN	Plumbago europaea (L.)
SYNONYMS	common leadwort
SPREAD	Asia, Europe
PLANT PARTS	herb, root
TEMPERATURE	230°C / 446°F
SUBSTANCES	bittering agent, acids
MEDICAL EFFECTS	anti-inflammatory, pain-relieving
FOLK MEDICINE	feeling comfortable, concentration, encounters, eroticizing effect, transformation, meditation

poet's jasmine

LATIN	Jasminum officinale (L.)
SYNONYMS	poet's jasmine, jessamine, white jasmine
SPREAD	Africa, Asia, Europe, North America, Oceania, South America
PLANT PARTS	blossoms, root
TEMPERATURE	210°C / 410°F
SUBSTANCES	essential oils
MEDICAL EFFECTS	good for the skin
FOLK MEDICINE	eroticizing effect, encounters

pomegranate

LATIN	Punica granatum (L.)
SYNONYMS	
SPREAD	Africa, Asia, Europe, North America
PLANT PARTS	leaves, fruit peel
TEMPERATURE	205°C / 401°F
SUBSTANCES	alkaloids, tanning agent, acids
MEDICAL EFFECTS	anti-carcinogenic
FOLK MEDICINE	concentration, encounters

porter´s licorice-root

LATIN	Ligusticum porteri (J.M. Coult. & Rose)
SYNONYMS	osha
SPREAD	North America, South America
PLANT PARTS	root
TEMPERATURE	220°C / 428°F
SUBSTANCES	alkaloids, essential oils, coumarins, saponins, acids
MEDICAL EFFECTS	anti-inflammatory, pain-relieving
FOLK MEDICINE	protection, eroticizing effect, meditation, encounters

potency wood

LATIN	Ptychopetalum olacoides (Benth.)
SYNONYMS	muira puama
SPREAD	South America
PLANT PARTS	wood, root
TEMPERATURE	225°C / 437°F
SUBSTANCES	essential oils
MEDICAL EFFECTS	aphrodisiac effect
FOLK MEDICINE	encounters, transformation

praying-hands

LATIN	Harungana madagascariensis (Lam. ex Poir.)
SYNONYMS	the dragon's blood tree, orange-milk tree, haronga
SPREAD	Africa
PLANT PARTS	leaves, bark
TEMPERATURE	195°C / 383°F
SUBSTANCES	essential oils, flavonoids
MEDICAL EFFECTS	antibacterial, digestive
FOLK MEDICINE	concentration, feeling comfortable, encounters, eroticizing effect

Prince-of-Wales feather

LATIN	Amaranthus hypochondriacus (L.)
SYNONYMS	Prince's-feather, amaranth
SPREAD	Africa, Asia, Europe, North America, Oceania, South America
PLANT PARTS	leaves, seeds
TEMPERATURE	225°C / 437°F
SUBSTANCES	flavonoids, minerals, acids
MEDICAL EFFECTS	antioxidant
FOLK MEDICINE	eroticizing effect, encounters, meditation, feeling comfortable, transformation, concentration

purple coneflower

LATIN	Echinacea purpurea (Moench)
SYNONYMS	eastern purple coneflower
SPREAD	Asia, Europe
PLANT PARTS	herb
TEMPERATURE	215°C / 419°F
SUBSTANCES	essential oils
MEDICAL EFFECTS	antiseptic, immuno-stimulating
FOLK MEDICINE	protection, concentration, encounters
NOTES	Is bred in Europe.

purple loosestrife

LATIN	Lythrum salicaria (L.)
SYNONYMS	purple lythrum, bouguet-violet, spiked loosestrife
SPREAD	Asia, Europe, North America, Oceania
PLANT PARTS	herb, root
TEMPERATURE	230°C / 446°F
SUBSTANCES	essential oils, flavonoids, tanning agent, glycosides, minerals
MEDICAL EFFECTS	antibacterial, dehydrating, diuretic, soporific
FOLK MEDICINE	protection, strengthening, transformation, concentration, feeling comfortable, eroticizing effect, encounters, meditation

purple passionflower

LATIN	Passiflora incarnata (L.)
SYNONYMS	may-pops, wild passionflower, apricot-vine
SPREAD	Asia, Europe, North America, South America
PLANT PARTS	herb
TEMPERATURE	220°C / 428°F
SUBSTANCES	essential oils, flavonoids, coumarins
MEDICAL EFFECTS	diuretic
FOLK MEDICINE	protection, transformation, encounters

Pyrenees star of Bethlehem

LATIN	Ornithogalum umbellatum (L.)
SYNONYMS	dove's-dung, nap-at-noon, garden star-of-Bethlehem, summer-snowflake, grass lily, eleven-o'clock lady
SPREAD	Europe, North America
PLANT PARTS	blossoms
TEMPERATURE	210°C / 410°F
SUBSTANCES	glycosides, saponins, slime
MEDICAL EFFECTS	hair growth-stimulating
FOLK MEDICINE	cleansing, transformation
NOTES	toxic

quassia wood

LATIN	Quassia amara (L.)
SYNONYMS	bitter-ash, bitter-wood, hombre grande, amargo
SPREAD	Africa, Asia, Oceania, South America
PLANT PARTS	wood
TEMPERATURE	250°C / 482°F
SUBSTANCES	essential oils, bittering agent, acids
MEDICAL EFFECTS	antipyretic, digestive
FOLK MEDICINE	protection, eroticizing effect, transformation, feeling comfortable

quince

LATIN	Cydonia oblonga (Mill.)
SYNONYMS	
SPREAD	Asia, Europe
PLANT PARTS	fruits, seeds
TEMPERATURE	220°C / 428°F
SUBSTANCES	essential oils, fatty oil, tanning agent, minerals, slime
MEDICAL EFFECTS	anti-inflammatory
FOLK MEDICINE	feeling comfortable, encounters, transformation

quinine

LATIN	Cinchona pubescens (Vahl), Quinquina pubescens (Kuntze)
SYNONYMS	quina, red cinchona, Jesuit's bark, Jesuit's powder
SPREAD	Africa, Asia, Europe, North America, Oceania, South America
PLANT PARTS	bark
TEMPERATURE	230°C / 446°F
SUBSTANCES	alkaloids, tanning agent
MEDICAL EFFECTS	antipyretic, pain-relieving
FOLK MEDICINE	concentration

red clover

LATIN	Trifolium pratense (L.)
SYNONYMS	
SPREAD	Africa, Asia, Europe, North America, Oceania, South America
PLANT PARTS	leaves
TEMPERATURE	220°C / 428°F
SUBSTANCES	essential oils, glycosides
MEDICAL EFFECTS	hormonal
FOLK MEDICINE	strengthening, encounters

red raspberry

LATIN	Rubus idaeus (L.)
SYNONYMS	European raspberry
SPREAD	Asia, Europe, North America, Oceania
PLANT PARTS	leaves
TEMPERATURE	220°C / 428°F
SUBSTANCES	flavonoids, tanning agent
MEDICAL EFFECTS	decongestant, calming, anti-inflammatory, diuretic, immuno-stimulating
FOLK MEDICINE	protection, strengthening, eroticizing effect, feeling comfortable, concentration, transformation

red sandalwood

LATIN	Pterocarpus santalinus (Buch.-Ham. ex Wall.)
SYNONYMS	red sanders, saunderswood
SPREAD	Asia
PLANT PARTS	wood
TEMPERATURE	230°C / 446°F
SUBSTANCES	essential oils
MEDICAL EFFECTS	antibacterial, aphrodisiac effect, anti-inflammatory
FOLK MEDICINE	strengthening, feeling comfortable, encounters, transformation

redroot sage

LATIN	Salvia miltiorrhiza (Bunge)
SYNONYMS	Chinese sage, danshen
SPREAD	Asia, Europe
PLANT PARTS	leaves
TEMPERATURE	230°C / 446°F
SUBSTANCES	flavonoids, tanning agent, acids, Steroide
MEDICAL EFFECTS	antibacterial, anti-carcinogenic
FOLK MEDICINE	eroticizing effect, concentration, feeling comfortable

rennet

LATIN	Withania somnifera (Dunal)
SYNONYMS	poison gooseberry, winter cherry, Indian winter cherry, ashwagandha, Indian ginseng
SPREAD	Africa, Asia, Europe
PLANT PARTS	root
TEMPERATURE	235°C / 455°F
SUBSTANCES	Steroide
MEDICAL EFFECTS	appetitstimulating, calming
FOLK MEDICINE	meditation

rhatany

LATIN	Krameria lappacea (Burdet & B.B. Simpson)
SYNONYMS	Peruvian rhatany
SPREAD	South America
PLANT PARTS	root
TEMPERATURE	250°C / 482°F
SUBSTANCES	tanning agent
MEDICAL EFFECTS	anti-inflammatory
FOLK MEDICINE	encounters

ribbed melilot

LATIN	Melilotus officinalis (Lam.)
SYNONYMS	melist, yellow melilot, common melilot, yellow sweet clover
SPREAD	Africa, Asia, Europe, North America, Oceania, South America
PLANT PARTS	herb
TEMPERATURE	240°C / 464°F
SUBSTANCES	flavonoids, glycosides, coumarins, acids, slime
MEDICAL EFFECTS	decongestant, anti-inflammatory, antispasmodic
FOLK MEDICINE	protection, strengthening, meditation, transformation, eroticizing effect, concentration

rosemary

LATIN	Rosmarinus officinalis (L.)
SYNONYMS	
SPREAD	Europe
PLANT PARTS	leaves
TEMPERATURE	225°C / 437°F
SUBSTANCES	essential oils, bittering agent, tanning agent, saponins, acids
MEDICAL EFFECTS	decongestant, antibacterial
FOLK MEDICINE	protection, cleansing, strengthening, concentration, eroticizing effect

roseroot

LATIN	Rhodiola rosea (L.)
SYNONYMS	golden root, western roseroot, Aaron's rod, arctic root, king's crown, orpin rose
SPREAD	Asia, Europe, North America
PLANT PARTS	herb
TEMPERATURE	210°C / 410°F
SUBSTANCES	essential oils, flavonoids, tanning agent, glycosides, minerals
MEDICAL EFFECTS	antidepressant, improving the ability to concentrate
FOLK MEDICINE	concentration, eroticizing effect

rosin

LATIN	Pinus (L.)
SYNONYMS	colophony, Greek pitch
SPREAD	Africa, Asia, Europe, North America, Oceania, South America
PLANT PARTS	resin
TEMPERATURE	250°C / 482°F (over 300°C / 572°F)
SUBSTANCES	essential oils
MEDICAL EFFECTS	anti-inflammatory, mucolytic
FOLK MEDICINE	cleansing, strengthening, meditation, feeling comfortable

Russian sage

LATIN	Perovskia atriplicifolia (Benth.)
SYNONYMS	
SPREAD	Asia
PLANT PARTS	herb
TEMPERATURE	220°C / 428°F
SUBSTANCES	essential oils
MEDICAL EFFECTS	anti-inflammatory, antipyretic
FOLK MEDICINE	strengthening, meditation, transformation

sacred bo tree

LATIN	Ficus religiosa (L.)
SYNONYMS	sacred fig, bodhi tree, pippala tree, ashwattha tree, peepul tree
SPREAD	Asia
PLANT PARTS	wood
TEMPERATURE	225°C / 437°F
SUBSTANCES	tanning agent, saponins
MEDICAL EFFECTS	anti-inflammatory
FOLK MEDICINE	strengthening, meditation

sacred lotus

LATIN	Nelumbo nucifera (Gaertn.)
SYNONYMS	bean of India, Oriental lotus, East Indian lotus, Hindu lotus
SPREAD	Asia, Europe, North America, Oceania
PLANT PARTS	root
TEMPERATURE	230°C / 446°F
SUBSTANCES	essential oils, acids
MEDICAL EFFECTS	blood pressure-reducing, constricting
FOLK MEDICINE	meditation, transformation

safflower

LATIN	Carthamus tinctorius (L.)
SYNONYMS	false saffron
SPREAD	Africa, Asia, Europe, North America, Oceania, South America
PLANT PARTS	blossoms
TEMPERATURE	210°C / 410°F
SUBSTANCES	acids
MEDICAL EFFECTS	antioxidant
FOLK MEDICINE	concentration, trance, dream, vision
NOTES	It is confused with real saffron and used as a red food colouring.

Saint John's wort

LATIN	Hypericum perforatum (L.)
SYNONYMS	perforate St John's-wort, eola-weed, goat-weed, klamath-weed, rosin-rose, Saint John's wart, Tipton's-weed
SPREAD	Africa, Asia, Europe, North America, Oceania, South America
PLANT PARTS	herb
TEMPERATURE	215°C / 419°F
SUBSTANCES	essential oils, bittering agent, flavonoids, tanning agent
MEDICAL EFFECTS	antidepressant
FOLK MEDICINE	protection, strengthening, eroticizing effect, concentration
NOTES	If possible, cut at lunchtime.

sal tree

LATIN	Shorea robusta (Gaertn.)
SYNONYMS	sakhua,shala tree, red balau
SPREAD	Asia
PLANT PARTS	resin
TEMPERATURE	235°C / 455°F (over 300°C / 572°F)
SUBSTANCES	essential oils
MEDICAL EFFECTS	constricting
FOLK MEDICINE	strengthening, encounters, trance, dream, vision

san-sho

LATIN	Zanthoxylum piperitum (DC.)
SYNONYMS	Japanese pricklyash,chopi, Japanese pepper, Korean pepper
SPREAD	Asia
PLANT PARTS	fruits, seeds
TEMPERATURE	210°C / 410°F
SUBSTANCES	essential oils
MEDICAL EFFECTS	anti-inflammatory
FOLK MEDICINE	cleansing, feeling comfortable, encounters

sandalwood

LATIN	Santalum album (L.)
SYNONYMS	santal, Indian sandalwood
SPREAD	Asia
PLANT PARTS	wood
TEMPERATURE	240°C / 464°F
SUBSTANCES	essential oils
MEDICAL EFFECTS	antibacterial, aphrodisiac effect, anti-inflammatory
FOLK MEDICINE	strengthening, feeling comfortable, encounters, meditation, transformation

savory

LATIN	Satureja hortensis (L.)
SYNONYMS	summer savory
SPREAD	Asia, Europe, North America
PLANT PARTS	leaves
TEMPERATURE	225°C / 437°F
SUBSTANCES	essential oils, tanning agent
MEDICAL EFFECTS	antibacterial, aphrodisiac effect, carminative
FOLK MEDICINE	concentration, meditation, feeling comfortable

saw palmetto

LATIN	Serenoa repens (Small)
SYNONYMS	
SPREAD	North America
PLANT PARTS	fruits
TEMPERATURE	200°C / 392°F
SUBSTANCES	essential oils, acids
MEDICAL EFFECTS	anti-inflammatory, hormonal
FOLK MEDICINE	feeling comfortable

scarlet pimpernel

LATIN	Anagallis arvensis (L.)
SYNONYMS	red pimpernel, red chickweed, poorman's barometer, poor man's weather-glass, shepherd's weather glass, blue-scarlet pimpernel, shepherd's clock
SPREAD	Africa, Asia, Europe, North America, Oceania, South America
PLANT PARTS	herb
TEMPERATURE	230°C / 446°F
SUBSTANCES	bittering agent, flavonoids, tanning agent, saponins
MEDICAL EFFECTS	antiseptic, pain-relieving
FOLK MEDICINE	strengthening, eroticizing effect, meditation, transformation

schefflera

LATIN	Rhamnus purshianus (DC.)
SYNONYMS	cascara buckthorn, chittem, chitticum, casara
SPREAD	North America
PLANT PARTS	bark
TEMPERATURE	225°C / 437°F
SUBSTANCES	anthranoids, glycosides
MEDICAL EFFECTS	laxative
FOLK MEDICINE	strengthening, feeling comfortable, concentration

scots pine

LATIN	Pinus sylvestris (L.)
SYNONYMS	Scotch pine
SPREAD	Asia, Europe
PLANT PARTS	resin, fruits, bark
TEMPERATURE	260°C / 500°F (over 300°C / 572°F)
SUBSTANCES	essential oils, bittering agent
MEDICAL EFFECTS	anti-inflammatory
FOLK MEDICINE	cleansing, strengthening, meditation, eroticizing effect, feeling comfortable, concentration

sea-buckthorn

LATIN	Hippophae rhamnoides (L.)
SYNONYMS	
SPREAD	Asia, Europe
PLANT PARTS	fruits, seeds
TEMPERATURE	200°C / 392°F
SUBSTANCES	essential oils, fatty oil, flavonoids, tanning agent, acids
MEDICAL EFFECTS	antibacterial, immuno-stimulating
FOLK MEDICINE	cleansing, eroticizing effect, meditation, transformation

serpentine wood

LATIN	Rauvolfia serpentina (Benth. ex Kurz)
SYNONYMS	Indian snakeroot
SPREAD	Africa, Asia, Oceania, South America
PLANT PARTS	leaves, herb, root
TEMPERATURE	220°C / 428°F
SUBSTANCES	alkaloids, essential oils
MEDICAL EFFECTS	calming
FOLK MEDICINE	meditation, eroticizing effect, transformation

sheep's sorrel

LATIN	Rumex acetosella (L.)
SYNONYMS	red sorrel, sour weed, field sorrel, sour dock
SPREAD	Africa, Asia, Europe, North America, Oceania, South America
PLANT PARTS	herb
TEMPERATURE	195°C / 383°F
SUBSTANCES	tanning agent, glycosides, minerals, acids
MEDICAL EFFECTS	laxative, immuno-stimulating
FOLK MEDICINE	eroticizing effect, encounters, concentration, meditation

shepherd's purse

LATIN	Capsella bursa-pastoris (Medik.), Thlaspi bursa-pastoris (L.)
SYNONYMS	shepherd's-purse
SPREAD	Asia, Europe
PLANT PARTS	herb
TEMPERATURE	220°C / 428°F
SUBSTANCES	flavonoids, tanning agent, glycosides, acids
MEDICAL EFFECTS	astringent
FOLK MEDICINE	meditation, trance, dream, vision

Siam benzoin

LATIN	Styrax tonkinensis (Craib ex Hartwich)
SYNONYMS	benzoin resin, gum benzoin, gum benjamin, styrax balsam, styrax resin
SPREAD	Asia
PLANT PARTS	resin
TEMPERATURE	230°C / 446°F (over 300°C / 572°F)
SUBSTANCES	essential oils, acids
MEDICAL EFFECTS	antibacterial, calming, antispasmodic, mucolytic
FOLK MEDICINE	strengthening, feeling comfortable, encounters, transformation

siamese ginger

LATIN	Alpinia galanga (Willd.), Maranta galanga (L.)
SYNONYMS	galangal, Thai galangal, blue ginger, Thai ginger
SPREAD	Asia, Europe
PLANT PARTS	root
TEMPERATURE	225°C / 437°F
SUBSTANCES	anthranoids, essential oils, flavonoids, tanning agent
MEDICAL EFFECTS	laxative, antibacterial, carminative, anti-inflammatory, antispasmodic, anti-carcinogenic
FOLK MEDICINE	cleansing, feeling comfortable, concentration, encounters, eroticizing effect

silver fir

LATIN	Abies alba
SYNONYMS	European silver fir
SPREAD	Europe
PLANT PARTS	resin, needles
TEMPERATURE	235°C / 455°F
SUBSTANCES	essential oils
MEDICAL EFFECTS	antimicrobiologic
FOLK MEDICINE	strengthening, encounters, concentration

silverweed

LATIN	Potentilla anserina (L.)
SYNONYMS	goose-grass, goose-tansy, silverweed cinquefoil
SPREAD	Asia, Europe, North America, Oceania
PLANT PARTS	herb, root
TEMPERATURE	240°C / 464°F
SUBSTANCES	bittering agent, flavonoids, tanning agent, glycosides, acids
MEDICAL EFFECTS	dehydrating, anti-inflammatory, antispasmodic, pain-relieving
FOLK MEDICINE	eroticizing effect, concentration, encounters, transformation, feeling comfortable, meditation

small scabious

LATIN	Scabiosa columbaria (L.)
SYNONYMS	great cheverell hill
SPREAD	Asia, Europe
PLANT PARTS	herb
TEMPERATURE	235°C / 455°F
SUBSTANCES	essential oils, flavonoids, tanning agent, glycosides, saponins
MEDICAL EFFECTS	invigorating
FOLK MEDICINE	encounters, transformation, eroticizing effect

smallflower hairy willowherb

LATIN	Epilobium parviflorum (Schreb.)
SYNONYMS	hoary willowherb
SPREAD	Africa, Asia, Europe, North America, Oceania, South America
PLANT PARTS	herb, root
TEMPERATURE	220°C / 428°F
SUBSTANCES	flavonoids, tanning agent, slime
MEDICAL EFFECTS	anti-inflammatory, constricting
FOLK MEDICINE	transformation, encounters, concentration, meditation

smooth hydrangea

LATIN	Hydrangea arborescens (L.)
SYNONYMS	wild hydrangea, sevenbark, American hydrangea, hills-of-snow
SPREAD	North America
PLANT PARTS	root
TEMPERATURE	240°C / 464°F
SUBSTANCES	essential oils, flavonoids, tanning agent, glycosides
MEDICAL EFFECTS	immuno-stimulating
FOLK MEDICINE	encounters, eroticizing effect

snowflake

LATIN	Lamium album (L.)
SYNONYMS	white nettle, white dead-nettle
SPREAD	Africa, Asia, Europe, North America, Oceania, South America
PLANT PARTS	herb
TEMPERATURE	210°C / 410°F
SUBSTANCES	essential oils, tanning agent, saponins, acids, slime
MEDICAL EFFECTS	anti-inflammatory
FOLK MEDICINE	strengthening, meditation, transformation, eroticizing effect, concentration

soapwort

LATIN	Saponaria officinalis (L.)
SYNONYMS	bouncingbet, crow soap, wild sweet William, soapweed
SPREAD	Asia, Europe, North America
PLANT PARTS	root
TEMPERATURE	220°C / 428°F
SUBSTANCES	saponins
MEDICAL EFFECTS	mucolytic, anti-carcinogenic
FOLK MEDICINE	protection, strengthening, eroticizing effect, feeling comfortable

Solomon's seal

LATIN	Polygonatum multiflorum (All.)
SYNONYMS	David's harp, ladder-to-heaven, Eurasian Solomon's seal
SPREAD	Asia, Europe, North America
PLANT PARTS	root
TEMPERATURE	215°C / 419°F
SUBSTANCES	essential oils
MEDICAL EFFECTS	diuretic
FOLK MEDICINE	encounters

sour cherry

LATIN	Prunus cerasus (L.)
SYNONYMS	tart cherry, dwarf cherry, pie cherry
SPREAD	Asia, Europe
PLANT PARTS	leaves, fruits
TEMPERATURE	220°C / 428°F
SUBSTANCES	flavonoids, tanning agent
MEDICAL EFFECTS	diuretic
FOLK MEDICINE	concentration, feeling comfortable

spiny restharrow

LATIN	Ononis spinosa (L.)
SYNONYMS	common restharrow
SPREAD	Europe
PLANT PARTS	root
TEMPERATURE	240°C / 464°F
SUBSTANCES	essential oils, flavonoids, tanning agent, glycosides, saponins
MEDICAL EFFECTS	anti-inflammatory, diuretic
FOLK MEDICINE	strengthening, encounters, eroticizing effect

spotted dog

LATIN	Pulmonaria officinalis (L.)
SYNONYMS	common lungwort, our lady's milk drops
SPREAD	Europe
PLANT PARTS	herb
TEMPERATURE	230°C / 446°F
SUBSTANCES	flavonoids, tanning agent, silica, minerals, saponins, acids, slime
MEDICAL EFFECTS	dehydrating, anti-inflammatory, mucolytic
FOLK MEDICINE	eroticizing effect, transformation, feeling comfortable, meditation, concentration

spring adonis

LATIN	Adonis vernalis (L.)
SYNONYMS	ox-eye, spring pheasant's eye, yellow pheasant's eye, false hellebore
SPREAD	Asia, Europe
PLANT PARTS	herb
TEMPERATURE	210°C / 410°F
SUBSTANCES	flavonoids, glycosides
MEDICAL EFFECTS	positively inotropic
FOLK MEDICINE	transformation, meditation, eroticizing effect
NOTES	toxic

stag's-horn moss

LATIN	Lycopodium clavatum (L.)
SYNONYMS	common club moss, buck-horn, running clubmoss, ground pine, wolf's foot clubmoss, coral-evergreen, elk-moss, running-pine, staghorn-evergreen, wolf's-claws
SPREAD	Africa, Asia, Europe, North America, South America
PLANT PARTS	herb
TEMPERATURE	230°C / 446°F
SUBSTANCES	alkaloids, acids
MEDICAL EFFECTS	anti-inflammatory, diuretic
FOLK MEDICINE	protection, eroticizing effect, transformation

star anise

LATIN	Illicium verum (Hook. f.)
SYNONYMS	Chinese star anise, badiam, Japanes anise
SPREAD	Africa, Asia, Oceania, South America
PLANT PARTS	fruits, seeds
TEMPERATURE	230°C / 446°F
SUBSTANCES	essential oils, tanning agent, saponins
MEDICAL EFFECTS	antispasmodic, mucolytic
FOLK MEDICINE	eroticizing effect, encounters, transformation

stinging nettle

LATIN	Urtica dioica (L.)
SYNONYMS	common nettle
SPREAD	Africa, Asia, Europe, North America, Oceania, South America
PLANT PARTS	leaves
TEMPERATURE	240°C / 464°F
SUBSTANCES	fatty oil, tanning agent, silica, minerals, acids
MEDICAL EFFECTS	antiseptic, stoffwechselstimulating
FOLK MEDICINE	protection, encounters, meditation

stone pine

LATIN	Pinus pinea (L.)
SYNONYMS	Italian stone pine, umbrella pine, parasol pine
SPREAD	Africa, Asia, Europe
PLANT PARTS	resin
TEMPERATURE	280°C / 536°F (over 300°C / 572°F)
SUBSTANCES	essential oils, acids
MEDICAL EFFECTS	anti-inflammatory, mucolytic
FOLK MEDICINE	cleansing, strengthening, meditation, feeling comfortable

strychnos

LATIN	Strychnos nux-vomica (L.) (L.)
SYNONYMS	nux vomica, poison nut, quaker buttons, strychnine tree
SPREAD	Asia, Oceania
PLANT PARTS	leaves, seeds
TEMPERATURE	225°C / 437°F
SUBSTANCES	alkaloids
MEDICAL EFFECTS	psychoactive
FOLK MEDICINE	trance, dream, vision , eroticizing effect, encounters
NOTES	highly toxic, paralyzing

styrax

LATIN	Styrax benzoin (Dryand.)
SYNONYMS	benjamin tree, loban, Sumatra benzoin tree
SPREAD	Asia
PLANT PARTS	resin
TEMPERATURE	250°C / 482°F (max. 260°C / 500°F)
SUBSTANCES	essential oils, acids
MEDICAL EFFECTS	antimicrobiologic , antioxidant , anti-inflammatory
FOLK MEDICINE	strengthening, feeling comfortable, encounters, meditation

sunpati

LATIN	Rhododendron lepidotum (Wall. ex G. Don)
SYNONYMS	
SPREAD	Asia
PLANT PARTS	leaves
TEMPERATURE	230°C / 446°F
SUBSTANCES	essential oils
MEDICAL EFFECTS	psychoactive
FOLK MEDICINE	encounters

sweet marjoram

LATIN	Origanum majorana (L.)
SYNONYMS	knotted marjoram, annual marjoram
SPREAD	Asia, Europe, North America
PLANT PARTS	leaves
TEMPERATURE	220°C / 428°F
SUBSTANCES	essential oils, bittering agent, tanning agent, saponins, acids
MEDICAL EFFECTS	calming
FOLK MEDICINE	cleansing, strengthening, eroticizing effect, feeling comfortable, concentration

sweet violet

LATIN	Viola odorata (L.)
SYNONYMS	wood violet, English violet, florist's violet, garden violet
SPREAD	Asia, Europe, North America, Oceania
PLANT PARTS	blossoms, root
TEMPERATURE	225°C / 437°F
SUBSTANCES	alkaloids, essential oils, flavonoids, slime
MEDICAL EFFECTS	anti-inflammatory
FOLK MEDICINE	meditation, eroticizing effect, encounters

sweet-flag

LATIN	Acorus calamus (L.)
SYNONYMS	calamus, beewort, flag root, muskrat root, pine root, rat root, sweet calomel, sweet cane, sweet myrtle, sweet rush, sweet sedge
SPREAD	Africa, Asia, Europe, North America
PLANT PARTS	root
TEMPERATURE	210°C / 410°F
SUBSTANCES	essential oils, bittering agent, acids, slime
MEDICAL EFFECTS	antibacterial, immuno-stimulating, antispasmodic, digestive
FOLK MEDICINE	cleansing, concentration, encounters, eroticizing effect

tangerine

LATIN	Citrus reticulata (Blanco)
SYNONYMS	mandarin orange, clementine orange
SPREAD	Africa, Asia, Oceania, South America
PLANT PARTS	leaves, peel
TEMPERATURE	220°C / 428°F
SUBSTANCES	essential oils, flavonoids, acids
MEDICAL EFFECTS	antioxidant
FOLK MEDICINE	concentration, eroticizing effect, feeling comfortable, meditation, encounters

tea

LATIN	Camellia sinensis (Kuntze)
SYNONYMS	tea shrub, tea tree, white tea, yellow tea, green tea, oolong, pu-erh tea, black tea
SPREAD	Africa, Asia, Oceania, South America
PLANT PARTS	leaves
TEMPERATURE	225°C / 437°F
SUBSTANCES	essential oils, flavonoids, tanning agent, minerals
MEDICAL EFFECTS	blood pressure-reducing, diuretic, immuno-stimulating
FOLK MEDICINE	strengthening, concentration

tea tree

LATIN	Melaleuca alternifolia (Cheel)
SYNONYMS	narrow-leaved tea-tree, snow-in-summer, narrow-leaved paperbark
SPREAD	Oceania
PLANT PARTS	leaves
TEMPERATURE	250°C / 482°F (max. 260°C / 500°F)
SUBSTANCES	essential oils
MEDICAL EFFECTS	antibacterial, antimycotic, antiseptic, antiviral, anti-inflammatory, immuno-stimulating, wound-healing
FOLK MEDICINE	cleansing, strengthening, concentration, transformation, meditation, eroticizing effect, feeling comfortable

tobacco

LATIN	Nicotiana tabacum (L.)
SYNONYMS	Virginia tobacco
SPREAD	Africa, Asia, Europe, North America, Oceania, South America
PLANT PARTS	leaves
TEMPERATURE	225°C / 437°F
SUBSTANCES	alkaloids
MEDICAL EFFECTS	psychoactive
FOLK MEDICINE	trance, dream, vision , eroticizing effect

tolu balsam

LATIN	Myroxylon balsamum (Harms), Toluifera balsamum (L.)
SYNONYMS	balsam tolu
SPREAD	South America
PLANT PARTS	resin
TEMPERATURE	260°C / 500°F (over 300°C / 572°F)
SUBSTANCES	essential oils, acids
MEDICAL EFFECTS	antibacterial, mucolytic
FOLK MEDICINE	strengthening, transformation, feeling comfortable, encounters
NOTES	The smoke is highly irritating to the respiratory tract and quickly triggers a severe cough.

tonka bean

LATIN	Dipteryx odorata (Willd.)
SYNONYMS	cumaru, kumaru, tonkin beans, tonquin beans
SPREAD	Africa
PLANT PARTS	beans, fruits, seeds
TEMPERATURE	205°C / 401°F
SUBSTANCES	essential oils, coumarins
MEDICAL EFFECTS	calming
FOLK MEDICINE	protection, eroticizing effect, feeling comfortable, encounters, meditation, trance, dream, vision

toothpick weed

LATIN	Ammi visnaga (Lam.)
SYNONYMS	toothpick-plant, bisnaga, toothpick ammi, toothpick cervil, Bishop's weed
SPREAD	Africa, Asia, Europe, North America, South America
PLANT PARTS	seeds
TEMPERATURE	215°C / 419°F
SUBSTANCES	essential oils, flavonoids, coumarins
MEDICAL EFFECTS	antispasmodic
FOLK MEDICINE	transformation, encounters

traveller's joy

LATIN	Clematis vitalba (L.)
SYNONYMS	old man's beard, evergreen clematis
SPREAD	Europe
PLANT PARTS	leaves, stems, root
TEMPERATURE	220°C / 428°F
SUBSTANCES	saponins, acids
MEDICAL EFFECTS	anti-inflammatory
FOLK MEDICINE	transformation, encounters, eroticizing effect, meditation

turmeric

LATIN	Curcuma longa (L.)
SYNONYMS	curcuma
SPREAD	Asia
PLANT PARTS	root
TEMPERATURE	210°C / 410°F
SUBSTANCES	essential oils
MEDICAL EFFECTS	anti-carcinogenic
FOLK MEDICINE	feeling comfortable
NOTES	Ayurvedic medicine

valerian

LATIN	Valeriana officinalis (L.)
SYNONYMS	garden valerian
SPREAD	Asia, Europe
PLANT PARTS	blossoms, root
TEMPERATURE	210°C / 410°F
SUBSTANCES	alkaloids, essential oils, bittering agent, tanning agent, acids
MEDICAL EFFECTS	calming, soporific
FOLK MEDICINE	protection, meditation, encounters, concentration

vanilla

LATIN	Vanilla planifolia (Andrews)
SYNONYMS	flat-leaved vanilla, Tahitian vanilla, West Indian vanilla
SPREAD	Africa, Asia, Oceania, South America
PLANT PARTS	fruits, seeds, pots
TEMPERATURE	250°C / 482°F
SUBSTANCES	essential oils, coumarins
MEDICAL EFFECTS	aphrodisiac effect, calming
FOLK MEDICINE	encounters, meditation

vanilla grass

LATIN	Hierochloe odorata (P.Beauv.)
SYNONYMS	sweet grass, manna grass, Mary's grass, holy grass, bison grass
SPREAD	Asia, Europe, North America
PLANT PARTS	leaves
TEMPERATURE	205°C / 401°F
SUBSTANCES	essential oils, coumarins
MEDICAL EFFECTS	antiseptic, calming
FOLK MEDICINE	protection, eroticizing effect, transformation, meditation

vervain

LATIN	Verbena officinalis (L.)
SYNONYMS	European vervain, common verbena
SPREAD	Africa, Asia, Europe, North America, Oceania, South America
PLANT PARTS	herb
TEMPERATURE	245°C / 473°F
SUBSTANCES	essential oils, bittering agent, tanning agent, glycosides, silica, slime
MEDICAL EFFECTS	calming
FOLK MEDICINE	cleansing, eroticizing effect, transformation

vetiver

LATIN	Vetiveria zizanioides (Nash), Chrysopogon zizanioides (Roberty), Andropogon zizanioides (Urb.)
SYNONYMS	khus, khuskhus vetiver
SPREAD	Africa, Asia, Oceania, South America
PLANT PARTS	root
TEMPERATURE	260°C / 500°F
SUBSTANCES	essential oils
MEDICAL EFFECTS	relaxing, immuno-stimulating
FOLK MEDICINE	encounters, meditation

wall germander

LATIN	Teucrium chamaedrys (L.)
SYNONYMS	
SPREAD	Africa, Asia, Europe
PLANT PARTS	herb
TEMPERATURE	215°C / 419°F
SUBSTANCES	essential oils, bittering agent, flavonoids, tanning agent, glycosides
MEDICAL EFFECTS	appetitstimulating, digestive
FOLK MEDICINE	eroticizing effect, transformation

walnut

LATIN	Juglans regia (L.)
SYNONYMS	Persian walnut, English walnut, Madeira-nut
SPREAD	Asia, Europe, North America
PLANT PARTS	leaves
TEMPERATURE	205°C / 401°F
SUBSTANCES	essential oils, bittering agent, fatty oil, flavonoids, tanning agent
MEDICAL EFFECTS	blood pressure-reducing, wound-healing
FOLK MEDICINE	concentration, feeling comfortable, meditation

watercress

LATIN	Nasturtium officinale (W.T. Aiton)
SYNONYMS	
SPREAD	Africa, Asia, Europe, North America, Oceania, South America
PLANT PARTS	herb
TEMPERATURE	200°C / 392°F
SUBSTANCES	essential oils, bittering agent, flavonoids, tanning agent, glycosides, minerals
MEDICAL EFFECTS	antibiotic, appetitstimulating, diuretic
FOLK MEDICINE	eroticizing effect, concentration

white bryony

LATIN	Bryonia alba (L.)
SYNONYMS	wild hop, false mandrake, wild vine, wild nep, tamus, ladies' seal, tetterbury
SPREAD	Africa, Asia, Europe
PLANT PARTS	root
TEMPERATURE	230°C / 446°F
SUBSTANCES	essential oils, bittering agent, tanning agent
MEDICAL EFFECTS	antidepressant, pain-relieving
FOLK MEDICINE	protection, strengthening, meditation, encounters, concentration, eroticizing effect
NOTES	toxic

white cedar

LATIN	Thuja occidentalis (L.)
SYNONYMS	northern whitecedar, eastern white-cedar, swamp cedar, arborvitae
SPREAD	Europe, North America
PLANT PARTS	needles
TEMPERATURE	250°C / 482°F
SUBSTANCES	essential oils, flavonoids, tanning agent, coumarins, minerals
MEDICAL EFFECTS	antiseptic, constricting
FOLK MEDICINE	strengthening, concentration, meditation

white dammar

LATIN	Vateria indica (L.)
SYNONYMS	dammar
SPREAD	Asia, Europe, Oceania
PLANT PARTS	resin
TEMPERATURE	255°C / 491°F (max. 280°C / 536°F)
SUBSTANCES	essential oils
MEDICAL EFFECTS	antiseptic
FOLK MEDICINE	strengthening, feeling comfortable, concentration, trance, dream, vision
NOTES	toxic

white quebracho

LATIN	Aspidosperma quebracho-blanco (Schltdl.)
SYNONYMS	kebrako, quebracho blancho
SPREAD	South America
PLANT PARTS	bark
TEMPERATURE	230°C / 446°F
SUBSTANCES	alkaloids, bittering agent
MEDICAL EFFECTS	antibacterial, diuretic, constricting
FOLK MEDICINE	eroticizing effect, concentration

white sage

LATIN	Salvia apiana (Jeps.)
SYNONYMS	bee sage, sacred sage, greasewood
SPREAD	North America
PLANT PARTS	leaves
TEMPERATURE	210°C / 410°F
SUBSTANCES	saponins, acids
MEDICAL EFFECTS	antiseptic
FOLK MEDICINE	strengthening, feeling comfortable, meditation

white turmeric

LATIN	Curcuma zedoaria (Roscoe), Amomum zedoaria (Christm.)
SYNONYMS	kentjur, zedoary
SPREAD	Asia, Europe, North America
PLANT PARTS	root
TEMPERATURE	225°C / 437°F
SUBSTANCES	essential oils, coumarins
MEDICAL EFFECTS	antispasmodic
FOLK MEDICINE	eroticizing effect, concentration

white willow

LATIN	Salix alba (L.)
SYNONYMS	
SPREAD	Africa, Asia, Europe
PLANT PARTS	leaves, bark
TEMPERATURE	215°C / 419°F
SUBSTANCES	tanning agent, glycosides, acids
MEDICAL EFFECTS	decongestant, astringent, anti-inflammatory, antipyretic, pain-relieving
FOLK MEDICINE	concentration, eroticizing effect, transformation, encounters, meditation, feeling comfortable
NOTES	One of the 4 holy Jewish plants (myrtle, date palm, willow, lemon).

wild chives

LATIN	Allium schoenoprasum (L.)
SYNONYMS	garlic chives, Chinese chives, schnittlauch
SPREAD	Asia, Europe, North America
PLANT PARTS	stems
TEMPERATURE	200°C / 392°F
SUBSTANCES	essential oils, flavonoids, glycosides, minerals, acids, slime
MEDICAL EFFECTS	antimicrobiologic , antimycotic, antiviral, appetitstimulating, blood pressure-reducing, anticoagulant, diuretic, mucolytic, digestive
FOLK MEDICINE	strengthening, meditation, encounters, eroticizing effect, concentration

wild garlic

LATIN	Allium ursinum (L.)
SYNONYMS	ramsons, buckrams, broad-leaved garlic, wood garlic, bear leek, bear's garlic, gipsy onion, hog~s garlic
SPREAD	Asia, Europe
PLANT PARTS	leaves
TEMPERATURE	220°C / 428°F
SUBSTANCES	essential oils, flavonoids, glycosides, acids, slime
MEDICAL EFFECTS	antimycotic, labor-inducing
FOLK MEDICINE	strengthening, concentration, eroticizing effect, feeling comfortable, meditation, encounters

wild liquorice

LATIN	Astragalus glycyphyllos (L.)
SYNONYMS	wild liquorice, wild licorice, liquorice milkvetch
SPREAD	Asia, Europe
PLANT PARTS	root
TEMPERATURE	220°C / 428°F
SUBSTANCES	essential oils, flavonoids, minerals, saponins, acids
MEDICAL EFFECTS	antiallergic
FOLK MEDICINE	protection, cleansing, strengthening, concentration, eroticizing effect, encounters
NOTES	Used as food additive E 413. One of the 50 most important substances in Chinese medicine.

wild pansy

LATIN	Viola tricolor (L.)
SYNONYMS	Johnny jump up, heartsease, heart's delight, tickle-my-fancy, Jack-jump-up-and-kiss-me, come-and-cuddle-me, three faces in a hood, love-in-idleness
SPREAD	Europe
PLANT PARTS	herb
TEMPERATURE	225°C / 437°F
SUBSTANCES	alkaloids, essential oils, tanning agent, acids, slime
MEDICAL EFFECTS	anti-inflammatory, mucolytic
FOLK MEDICINE	protection, cleansing, eroticizing effect, meditation, concentration
NOTES	protected plant

wild quinine

LATIN	Parthenium integrifolium (L.)
SYNONYMS	American feverfew, eastern parthenium
SPREAD	North America
PLANT PARTS	herb
TEMPERATURE	240°C / 464°F
SUBSTANCES	tanning agent
MEDICAL EFFECTS	wound-healing
FOLK MEDICINE	meditation

wild strawberry

LATIN	Fragaria vesca (L.)
SYNONYMS	woodland strawberry, alpine strawberry, European strawberry, sow-teat strawberry
SPREAD	Africa, Asia, Europe, North America, Oceania, South America
PLANT PARTS	leaves, root
TEMPERATURE	245°C / 473°F
SUBSTANCES	essential oils, flavonoids, tanning agent, silica
MEDICAL EFFECTS	antibacterial
FOLK MEDICINE	concentration, eroticizing effect, feeling comfortable

wood sanicle

LATIN	Sanicula europaea (L.)
SYNONYMS	sanicle
SPREAD	Africa, Asia, Europe
PLANT PARTS	herb
TEMPERATURE	225°C / 437°F
SUBSTANCES	essential oils, bittering agent, flavonoids, tanning agent, saponins
MEDICAL EFFECTS	appetitstimulating, astringent, anti-inflammatory, wound-healing
FOLK MEDICINE	eroticizing effect, meditation, feeling comfortable, transformation, concentration

woodland figwort

LATIN	Scrophularia nodosa (L.)
SYNONYMS	common figwort
SPREAD	Asia, Europe, North America
PLANT PARTS	herb, root
TEMPERATURE	230°C / 446°F
SUBSTANCES	essential oils, flavonoids, saponins, acids
MEDICAL EFFECTS	diuretic, wound-healing
FOLK MEDICINE	protection, transformation, encounters, feeling comfortable, concentration, eroticizing effect, meditation

woodruff

LATIN	Galium odoratum (Scop.)
SYNONYMS	sweetscented bedstraw, sweet woodruff, waldmeister
SPREAD	Asia, Europe, North America
PLANT PARTS	herb
TEMPERATURE	220°C / 428°F
SUBSTANCES	glycosides, coumarins, acids
MEDICAL EFFECTS	antiseptic, calming, cleansing, diuretic, antispasmodic
FOLK MEDICINE	strengthening, eroticizing effect, meditation, transformation, encounters, concentration

woundwort

LATIN	Anthyllis vulneraria (L.)
SYNONYMS	common kidneyvetch, kidney vetch, lady's-fingers
SPREAD	Africa, Europe
PLANT PARTS	herb
TEMPERATURE	205°C / 401°F
SUBSTANCES	flavonoids, tanning agent, saponins
MEDICAL EFFECTS	stimulating, antibacterial, astringent, diuretic, cough suppressant, wound-healing
FOLK MEDICINE	meditation, transformation, feeling comfortable, eroticizing effect, concentration

yarrow

LATIN	Achillea millefolium (L.)
SYNONYMS	common yarrow
SPREAD	Africa, Asia, Europe, North America, Oceania, South America
PLANT PARTS	blossoms
TEMPERATURE	220°C / 428°F
SUBSTANCES	essential oils, bittering agent, flavonoids, tanning agent
MEDICAL EFFECTS	appetitstimulating, immuno-stimulating, digestive
FOLK MEDICINE	protection, trance, dream, vision , encounters, transformation, feeling comfortable, meditation

yellow gentian

LATIN	Gentiana lutea (L.)
SYNONYMS	bitter root, bitterwort, centiyane, genciana
SPREAD	Europe
PLANT PARTS	root
TEMPERATURE	220°C / 428°F
SUBSTANCES	bittering agent, tanning agent, acids, slime
MEDICAL EFFECTS	appetitstimulating , digestive
FOLK MEDICINE	cleansing, eroticizing effect, concentration

yerba de la pastora

LATIN	Salvia divinorum (Epling & Játiva)
SYNONYMS	sage of the diviners, seer's sage, salvia
SPREAD	South America
PLANT PARTS	herb
TEMPERATURE	220°C / 428°F
SUBSTANCES	minerals
MEDICAL EFFECTS	psychoactive
FOLK MEDICINE	trance, dream, vision , concentration
NOTES	Difficult to find in Europe and prohibited in some countries.

yerba mate

LATIN	Ilex paraguariensis (A. St.-Hil.)
SYNONYMS	
SPREAD	South America
PLANT PARTS	leaves
TEMPERATURE	215°C / 419°F
SUBSTANCES	alkaloids, essential oils, tanning agent, acids
MEDICAL EFFECTS	stimulating, digestive
FOLK MEDICINE	protection, trance, dream, vision , meditation, concentration

yerba santa

LATIN	Eriodictyon californicum (Torr.)
SYNONYMS	holi herb, mountain balm, consumptive's weed, bear weed
SPREAD	North America
PLANT PARTS	herb
TEMPERATURE	210°C / 410°F
SUBSTANCES	essential oils, flavonoids
MEDICAL EFFECTS	anti-inflammatory
FOLK MEDICINE	protection, meditation, transformation
NOTES	Cancels the taste sensation for "bitter".

Index

Books

Title	Author	ISBN
Das Buch vom Räuchern	Fischer-Rizzi, Susanne, Ebenhoch, Peter	978-3-03800-142-3
Das grosse Buch vom Räuchern	Susanne Fischer-Rizzi	978-3-03800-429-5
Das große Buch vom Räuchern	Franz X. J. Huber, Anja Schmidt	978-3-8434-3028-9
Das große kleine Buch: Räuchern mit Kräutern und Harzen	Barbara Haider, Hans Haider	978-3-7104-0014-8
Der Kosmos-Heilpflanzenführer: über 600 Heil- und Giftpflanzen Europas	Schönfelder, Ingrid, und Peter Schönfelder	978-3-440-14673-6
Einfach räuchern	Susanne Berk	978-3-86728-201-7
Flora Helvetica	Konrad Lauber, Gerhart Wagner	3-258-06313-3
Heilpflanzen für die Gesundheit: 333 Pflanzen - neues und überliefertes Heilwissen ; Pflanzenheilkunde, Homöopathie und Aromakunde.	Puhle, Annekatrin, Jürgen Trott-Tschepe, und Birgit Möller.	978-3-440-12235-8
Incense and Incense Rituals: Healing Ceremonies for Spaces of Subtle	Thomas Kinkele	978-0914955764
Incense: Its Ritual Significance, Use and Preparation	Leo Vinci	978-0850302110
Incense: Rituals, Mystery, Lore	Hyams, G.	978-0-8118-3993-8
Legends of Incense, Herb, and Oil Magic	De Claremont, L	978-0-9961471-1-8
Magic with incense and powders	Riva, A.	978-0-943832-11-1
Mein Räucherkistchen	Christine Fuchs	978-3-440-14893-8

Title	Author	ISBN
Psychologie des Räucherns	Thomas Kinkele	978-3-89385-623-7
Räuchern im Rhythmus der Jahreskreises	Christine Fuchs	978-3-440-14571-5
Räuchern in Winterzeit und Raunächten	Christine Fuchs	978-3-440-13328-6
Räuchern mit heimischen Kräutern	Marlis Bader	978-3-442-21811-0
Räuchern mit heimischen Pflanzen	Christine Fuchs	978-3-440-12610-3
Räuchern mit Kräutern	Roman Verster	978-3-86733-264-4
Räuchern mit Kräutern von Wiesen und Weiden	Tamara Hayndal	978-3-7357-8230-4
Räuchern, Räucherstoffe und Rituale	Zora Gienger	978-3-89901-436-5
Räucherstoffe und Räucherstäbchen	Georg Huber	978-3-89767-858-3
The complete incense book	Susanne Fischer-Rizzi	978-0-8069-9987-6
The Incense Bible: Plant Scents That Transcend World Culture, Medicine, and Spirituality	Kerry Hughes	978-0789021700
Wohnen in guter Energie	Marlis Bader	978-3-466-34496-3

Internet references

Title, Land	Date	Link
Botanica, CH	2018	http://www.botanica.ch/cms/en/
FDA Poisonous Plant Database, USA	2018	https://www.accessdata.fda.gov/scripts/plantox/
Flowers of India, India	2018	http://www.flowersofindia.net/index.html
Heilpflanzen-Experten, DE	2018	http://heilpflanzen-experten.de
Katuschka´s Celticgarden, DE	2018	http://www.celticgarden.de
Kräuterlexikon - 700 Heilpflanzen, DE	2018	http://heilkraeuter.de/lexikon/index.htm
MedFacts Natural Products A-Z Index, USA	2018	https://www.drugs.com/npc/
PharmaWiki, CH	2018	http://www.pharmawiki.ch/wiki/
Phytodoc, DE	2018	http://www.phytodoc.de/heilpflanzen
Phytokompass, DE	2018	http://phytokompass.de/heilpflanzen/
Plantnet	2018	https://identify.plantnet-project.org/
U of A, USA	2018	http://www.uaex.edu/yard-garden/resource-library/
Wikipedia, DE Die freie Enzyklopädie	2018	https://de.wikipedia.org/
Wikipedia, EN	2018	https://en.wikipedia.org/